Doing Single Well
A Guide to Living, Loving and Dating
Without Compromise

BY GEMMA CRIBB

THE AUTHOR

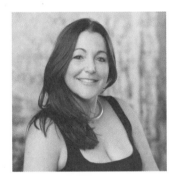

Gemma Cribb (B Psych (Hons), M Psychol (Clin)) is a Clinical Psychologist working in private practice in Sydney, Australia. She is an avid learner and has trained in many therapeutic approaches. Gemma has specialised in couples' therapy, relationships and sexuality. In the last ten years of treating people in Sydney's CBD, she has become particularly interested in the plight of single women.

As a happily single woman herself she became interested in what it took to 'Do Single Well' and enjoy single life despite the pessimistic views often encountered in the media and with concerned friends and family. To this end she began a blog addressing the most common areas single women struggle with, and academic research in the area.

Outside of blogging (www.gemmacribb.com), her clinical work and whatever crazy thing she is currently studying, you would generally find her at yoga, on a date, going for long walks between cafés or out for a wine with her friends.

First published in Great Britain 2018 by Trigger

The Foundation Centre
Navigation House, 48 Millgate, Newark
Nottinghamshire NG24 4TS UK

www.triggerpublishing.com

British Library Cataloguing in Publication Data

A CIP catalogue record for this book is available upon request from the British Library

ISBN: 978-1-912478-05-7

This book is also available in the following Audio and e-Book formats:

MOBI: 978-1-912478-08-8
EPUB: 978-1-912478-06-4
PDF: 978-1-912478-07-1
AUDIO: 978-1-912478-80-4

Cover design and typeset by Fusion Graphic Design Ltd

Project Management by Out of House Publishing

Printed and bound in Great Britain by Bell & Bain, Glasgow

Paper from responsible sources

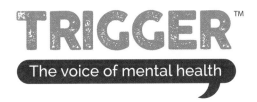

www.triggerpublishing.com

Thank you for purchasing this book.
You are making an incredible difference.

Proceeds from all Trigger books go directly to
The Shaw Mind Foundation, a global charity that focuses
entirely on mental health. To find out more about
The Shaw Mind Foundation, visit **www.shawmindfoundation.org**

MISSION STATEMENT

Our goal is to make help and support available for every
single person in society, from all walks of life.
We will never stop offering hope. These are our promises.

Trigger and The Shaw Mind Foundation

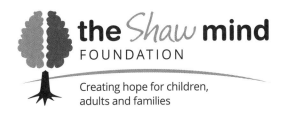

Creating hope for children,
adults and families

CONTENTS

PART IV
A FRESH APPROACH TO DATING

INTRODUCTION

WHY THIS BOOK

This book is not another dating manual. It is not filled with rules that sound good in theory, but are impossible or unhelpful in practice. It is also not a book that tries to teach you how to understand men, as if they are some unknown alien species. It will not give you an exhaustive historical account of the experiences of single women (check out *All the Single Ladies (2016)* by Rebecca Traister, it's great!). I will not be telling you to celebrate being single if you are desperate to be in a relationship. Nor will I give you advice to "love yourself first," without any practical ideas of how to do that!

What this book aims to do is acknowledge and support the lived experience of single women today. It was inspired by the many stories that my clients in my work as a Clinical Psychologist, friends, and the women who participated in my research have shared, as well as my own personal experience of *Doing Single Well*. I have included direct quotes and stories that honor the struggles and the wisdom of the single women that I've helped. However, to maintain anonymity, all names have been altered (except mine)!

Unfortunately, most of the single women I've met have shared stories about times in their lives where they have had low self-esteem, anxiety, and depression related to being single. It seems that whether single women are actively dating or not, we are vulnerable to losing our enjoyment of being single, and feeling unable to change our circumstances. These feelings can start a vicious cycle which makes us less likely to form a healthy relationship.

Being a single woman in our society today is tough. Unlike the term "bachelorette" which is generally used to describe single women who are about to be married, being "single" is a term used to describe people with no current marital prospects. We live in a culture that still sees "happily ever after" as being in a couple. Being single isn't just stigmatized, it is often seen as a failure. Whereas a bachelorette is more entitled to feel confident and self-assured and to cherish, even exploit, her time-limited independence, single women are encouraged to fear their biological clock and loneliness. They are subtly pushed to doubt their attractiveness and to work hard to improve themselves. To "settle" if Mr. Right doesn't show up.

I believe that it is possible to Do Single Well: For a single woman to feel self-confident, to feel attractive without self-improvement, to feel fulfilled and enjoy her life, and, if she wants a partner, to wait for one who is right for her.

No matter where you are on this journey, my deepest hope is that this book will help you join the growing ranks of single women who are satisfied single and, if they choose to date, delight in doing so!

This book will help you understand your experiences of being single today by dipping into a selection of the cultural and historical events that have shaped those experiences. You will be taken through a psychological perspective on what makes single women vulnerable to depression and anxiety, and you will be given practical tools for dealing with these thoughts, feelings, and situations if they occur for you. Most importantly, this book will guide you in the essential work of staying true to yourself, and being honest about your feelings, so you can be happy in your single life and have the best chances of finding your Mr. Right (if that is what you want).

Because part of Doing Single Well is finding a tribe or community of like-minded people, we have established a Facebook page @doingsinglewell. On Instagram we encourage you to use the hashtag #doingsinglewell to post your thoughts on the content of this book and any of the activities I recommend.

Although I will make every effort to interact with single women as much as possible in social media land, part of my own Doing Single Well means limiting my screen time, so please protect yourself:

- Don't post anything that makes you feel too exposed or vulnerable

- Don't post anything that requires urgent attention

- Social media is not an adequate substitute for therapy – please get some help if you need it

- Please disguise the identities of anyone you speak about. Be the politeness you would like to experience in the world!

Although this book is written from a heterosexual female orientation, I do invite single men, and people of all sexual orientations to take and adapt what ideas and practices they feel are relevant to them. In a society where the couple still reigns supreme, I would be delighted if the perspectives and tools I describe can improve the experiences of as many singles as possible.

PART I

'WHY ARE THERE SO MANY SINGLE WOMEN THESE DAYS?'

Being single and what that comes to mean for us does not happen in isolation. Our day-to-day lives are all influenced by a multitude of factors that are generally outside of our conscious awareness, including historical, political, and cultural developments. This section will help us understand the lived experience of single women currently, with reference to these contextual factors.

CHAPTER 1

WHY ARE YOU SINGLE?

'Why are you single?'

It is the dreaded question ... even if they don't ask, you *know* it's what they're wondering. What's worse, it's the same question you've found yourself wondering with every new guy you date. Because, all the good ones are taken, right?! Therefore, if he is single there *must* be something wrong with him, even if you can't see what it is yet. It's like the end-of-season bargain-basement bin. Only the junk nobody wants gets left behind. Anything worth having would have been snapped up when it first hit the store. So, if you are single, that must mean ...

ABSOLUTELY NOTHING!

There are many, many reasons for people "going on the market" at different ages and stages. But it always amazes me how many fabulous single women find fault with themselves (and with the guys they date!) using this kind of dubious logic. Of course, the dating rulebooks and airbrushed magazine covers don't help. Being asked the dreaded question at every family function, every reunion, every dinner party – in fact every time you are around groups of couples (which can be most of the time) – certainly doesn't help!

For many ladies, being single is not a conscious choice that we can identify a "why" for. It's not like 'Why did you choose to holiday in the Bahamas?' It's not even a preference we identify with. It's not like 'why do you have milk in your tea?' We *don't* actively choose or prefer it. Yet the question keeps being asked, and single women keep having to come up with some half-baked answer for it.

Unfortunately, if we think we are too ugly, too fat, too old, too boring, too tall, too serious, too light-hearted, too shy, too loud, too smart, too stupid, too successful, too lazy, too picky, too needy, too cool … and if we google hard enough, we'll always find some rot to support our self-hate.

Moreover, every friend and relative will have their own personal theory as to what men find attractive, and what we are doing wrong. And you can bet they'll be more than happy to share it with us at the first opportunity! But no matter how much the article we're reading feels like it was written about us, no matter how long our friend has known us, *no one* knows why we are still single. No one has been with us, in our head, on our dates, living through our experiences the whole time.

Now, it is certainly possible that you are tripping yourself up in the dating world. There are as many ways that single women sabotage their own efforts to find a partner as there are whys. This is something we'll spend a bit of time exploring later in the book. However, what I am saying is that this is not the full picture. And I should know …

GEM'S STORY

So, why am I single?

It's not because I'm ugly or fat. Like Bridget Jones, it's not because 'underneath my clothes my entire body is covered in scales.' It's not because I don't get out. My poor neglected fridge rarely sees groceries, I eat out so much. I'm not a nervous dater. In fact, I've been accused of liking dating too much for my own good! I'm not boring, stupid, frigid, or psycho.

I'm just single.

It's not that I always dreamed of being single. Like every child of the 80s I watched way too much Disney, and kind of assumed that when I grew up I'd meet my "handsome prince" (who would preferably look like *The Little Mermaid's* Prince Eric) and we would live happily ever after.

As I grew up, I also developed an awareness that there were certain things I wanted to do before I found my prince. Traveling, partying, dating, getting a university education, and beginning my career seemed important prerequisites for a well-lived life, and so I was in no rush to settle down.

In my 20s I threw myself into my studies and traveled the world. I had a fabulous time with fun-loving friends, and built my career and my business. I dated when I felt like it, and had a few lovely boyfriends.

Then, gradually, my heterosexual friends began to get married. One by one, the wedding cakes were cut and bouquets were thrown into an ever-decreasing gaggle of single ladies. Being part of this shrinking minority got me thinking hard about whether marriage was something I wanted.

My parents are joined in miserable matrimony until death do they part, and I still don't have a close real-life role model of a long-lasting happily married couple. My baby sister, 13 years my junior, was a terror toddler, and so I have long been cured of any starry-eyed delusions of how blissful motherhood might be.

Moreover, my life is awesome. My time is mine. I can do what I want, when I want. As my internet dating profile reads, I am a 'genuinely happy person, truly grateful for the life I lead. I have a job that I love, that allows me to work for myself, surround myself with great people, and affords me all the pretty things that I could want … I live in a great part of what I consider to be the best city in the world. I have fabulous friends, interests I indulge, and I travel at least yearly,' … I even get to write a book in my spare time – how cool is that?! Do I even want a partner?

In truth, the answer to that question still changes like the tide. Sometimes yes. Sometimes no. During my "yes" periods I meet lovely men and have a lot of fun. During my "no" periods I stop dating and have a lot of fun. Some people might say I go out of my way to choose unavailable men. Other's might say I "just haven't found the right one." My closest friends have accused me of not getting over "the one who got away." Maybe all of these are true in part. But if you're asking me now, 'Gem, why are you still single?' I think the most honest answer is:

This is where life has led me.

I have neither hunted down a relationship nor pushed it away. I feel that, like a rudderless boat, my present circumstances merely reflect where the current of the opportunities I've had has taken me.

And tomorrow, I might end up on relationship shores … who knows? All I know is that either way, my aim will be to remain happy and fulfilled, and to have an exciting journey. That, to me, is Doing Single Well.

HETERONORMATIVITY AND SINGLISM

To understand why you are single, you must first understand why the question is asked in the first place. I mean, you don't often get asked why you went to school, or why you sleep at night, do you? People seem particularly interested in our choices, particularly in the areas of our lives where we don't follow the norm (or their idea of it anyway!). There are norms in all areas of life, and although they might vary somewhat from culture to culture and subculture to subculture, most cultures across the globe perceive heterosexuality and the narrative of growing up, getting married, and having babies as a strong and enduring norm.

Heteronormativity is a term that was popularized by Michael Warner (1991). It refers to the idea that a relationship between one man and one woman is the normal form of sexuality. Singlism is the stereotyping, discrimination, and stigmatization of people who are single. Bella De Paulo first coined this term in 2005 and her later book *Singled Out: How Singles Are Stereotyped, Stigmatized and Ignored and Still Manage to Live Happily Ever After* (2006) is a great read if you are looking to explore the concept in greater depth.

Heteronormativity and singlism are present in all societies in the Western world. However, the more specific expectations and pressures that you will face can vary depending on the community and culture you live in. The following story exemplifies what the heteronormative ideal is for a middle-class woman in Sydney, Australia, where I live:

'Everything in my life has gone like clockwork until recently. I graduated high school and got into uni. I deferred for a year and did a gap year in the UK. I had a lot of fun traveling and meeting new people, knowing that I'd be coming home to get stuck in to my studies. In my first year back home, I met Mark. He was my first love, but I always knew we were too young to get married. I was heartbroken when we broke up, but I'd also just started my career and was keen to make a good impression.

I dated, but I didn't really have time for a serious relationship. My parents had just started to worry that I was focused on the wrong things and that I should get to finding "Mr. Right" when I went to my best friend's engagement party and met Steve. I was 27 years old, the perfect age to think about settling down' – Jennie, 37 years old.

This example reveals many of the life stages and goals that Jennie has internalized, growing up in her culture and socio-economic group. As we can see, Jennie feels it is normal and expected that she should finish school and do further study, with a view to having a career. However, you'll also notice that there are expectations that she shouldn't get married "too young" and that she should travel and "have fun." In cultures like Jennie's, getting married too young is seen as just as problematic as not getting married at all. You'll also notice the presumption of heterosexuality in the way Jennie speaks about her relationships and her parent's expectations.

Although not in her description, there may be other socially endorsed details that Jennie would assume are normal and "right." For example, she might feel it "too desperate" to ask a guy out, feeling she must wait to be asked. She might feel like she should have sex before marriage, but might also be conscious of not having sex with too many men for fear of being labeled a slut. She might feel pressure to pay attention to her appearance and not emphasize her brains or career achievements, in case men find her too intimidating. She might be discouraged from proposing marriage, instead needing to wait to be proposed to. She might feel pressure to wear an engagement and wedding ring. She might feel pressure to have babies. All these ideas and more can come through in our societies' messages to us as women.

Women that abide by this "normal" life course are generally approved of, and considered "on track." Women who deviate from this path in any way experience resistance from the people and the structures in their society. From gendered bathrooms to holiday package deals, from tables for two at restaurants to family tax or health insurance breaks, from the layout of seats on a bus to the quantity of milk in a carton, we live in a world where the expectation to couple is so pervasive that it is built into the fabric of society. It is so commonplace that it is almost invisible.

On top of this invisible messaging, we can add in all the overt stuff ... All the fairy tales, chick lit, and the rom-coms, all the couples pictured on billboards and on TV, all the tabloid articles on how to catch a man, and who's marrying who, and all the industries selling products to enhance your attractiveness and sex appeal. We are exposed to it all on a daily basis, and it is this layering and repetition of unvaried messaging that lays the groundwork for the sense of inadequacy and shame we feel whenever anyone asks, 'why are you single?'

What is more, if you identify as being in another marginalized group, like many of the ladies I interviewed did, it seems that the discrimination you may face is compounded. As De Paulo says, 'The pity that singles put up with is just not in the same league as the outright hatred conveyed to blacks by shameless racists or the unbridled disgust heaped upon gay men or lesbians by homophobes' (2006, p10) ... but it doesn't help matters.

DOING SINGLE WELL: MAKING THE INVISIBLE VISIBLE

For the next day pay attention to the heteronormative pressure and signs of singlism around you. Whenever you watch TV, read a book, listen to songs, catch a bus, go shopping, visit a restaurant, cinema ... look out for signs that a male / female couple is considered the norm. Take note of any comments made to you that might presume heteronormativity and convey singlism, and any imagery or stories that convey an idea of what the hetero couple's life is supposed to look like where you come from. Write your own "ideal" life course based on the expectations you feel are implicit in your society. Post your photos on Instagram with the hashtag #doingsinglewell or add your story to our Facebook page @doingsinglewell

DOING SINGLE WELL: HAPPILY EVER AFTER HYPNOSIS

Think back to your favorite movie or book from your childhood or teenage years. What did the storyline assume was "normal"? What messages might you have unconsciously – almost hypnotically – picked up from the storyline and themes about dating and relationships? As a little girl I used to love the "makeover" theme in movies like Disney's *Cinderella* and *Pretty Woman* starring Julia Roberts and Richard Gere. On reflection, what I *don't* love is the message that a woman has to undergo a physical transformation – become beautiful and well-dressed – to be good wife material! Post your favorite childhood stories and what messages they convey on our Facebook page @doingsinglewell

A WOMAN'S WORTH

A woman's worth has been tied to her marriageability for as long as we can deduce, and across cultures. As early as the 5th century BC we see references in Homer's *Iliad*, one of the earliest written works of Western literature, to a daughter being given in marriage to Achilles in order to secure an alliance. He could 'choose for himself twenty Trojan women, the most beautiful after Helen. Then, if we return to Argos, he shall have my daughter to wife ... I have three daughters ... any one of these he shall have without bride price ... and I will give her a dowry greater than any man gave to a daughter' (*Lliad* 121–22). The commodification of women as transactable marriage partners (and the less suitable ones for slaves and sex) seems to have occurred from the earliest time in civilization.

In modern weddings it is still common for a bride's father to "give her away" and in many cultures, arranged marriages, bride prices, and dowries are still customary. Yet, even in cultures where it is now customary to marry for love, not as a financial, social, or political arrangement, this notion that only the good and worthy are selected for marriage remains a popular bias. Is it any wonder that we still assume that our wedding day should be "the happiest day of our lives"?

Perhaps this is because up until relatively recently, a woman couldn't be educated and provide for herself; she was dependent on her father, and later her husband, for survival. The inequality in financial independence meant that until recently, women who did not inherit money were seen as a relative burden to be taken on and cared for by men, creating a power differential where a woman's security relied on a man to choose her. Even wealthy women such as Elizabeth I, "the Virgin Queen" who ruled England from 1558 to 1603, received great pressure to marry. The Virgin Queen notably never succumbed to such pressure, but most women without fortune or property could not afford to be so choosy.

The concept of romantic love was first popularized in Western culture in the Middle Ages between knights and the high-status women they served. Originally known as "courtly love," this relationship of caring and emotional closeness was not one that resulted in marriage. Marriage at this time was still reserved for the purpose of political, financial, or social alliances. As illustrated in Shakespeare's famous *Romeo and Juliet*, published in 1597, falling in love was not considered an adequate reason for marriage, and marriage for love alone was opposed.

Jane Austen writes about romantic love at the end of the 18th century. Yet, as with Shakespeare's work, her novels still suggest women were a commodity that could be comparatively valued, and to marry for love alone was a "fool's choice." A man would only court a wife who was attractive, accomplished, and preferably came with a large fortune. In *Pride and Prejudice* (1813, Chapter 3) Mr. Darcy says about Lizzie, 'She is tolerable I suppose, but not handsome enough to tempt me; I'm in no humor at present to give consequence to young ladies who are slighted by other men.' Although the Bennet heroines eventually married for love, as fortuneless women, their happy endings still all came about solely through marriage. It wasn't just their survival; the esteem of others, their social standing and their worth as a person were all solidified if they were chosen by men to be wives.

Nowadays, when a great many more women are able to financially support themselves, it seems we still see partner selection in terms of a "market place." This may be due to the very nature of monogamy where only being able to choose one sexual partner begets a challenge or competition to secure the "best" partner we can. There is opportunity cost in staying with, or committing to, someone who is not "right" as monogamy means we can't then pursue another, potentially better partner. By inference the partners that aren't "snapped up" and instead "left on the shelf" (notice the marketplace turns of phrase) must therefore be defective.

GOOD WIFE MATERIAL

So, if back in Jane Austen's days "good wife material" was someone who was wealthy and pretty, and could play the pianoforte, what makes for good wife material now? Who do people pick when they can pick for love?

I caution you *not* to look this up. In fact, I urge you to take most of the research you read about with a grain of salt. You'll find as many theories and research papers as you do "experts" on the matter. It's all so confusing and almost impossible to separate what to believe from what is rubbish. My horror at the self-defeating nonsense that is out there was part of the motivation for me putting this book together! So, please be very selective when it comes to what you read in the dating arena, and don't be afraid to challenge this book too! Take on board any perspective that propels you in a positive, constructive, self-affirmatory direction and ignore anything that make you feel hopeless, helpless, or disillusioned.

Let's confront one of those popular theories and see how it stacks up: it's said that across cultures, men choose women for youth and beauty while women choose men for status and security. The common explanation is that for survival of the species, women need men who can provide for them and their babies, and men need women who are fertile and can give them babies! It is an intriguing theory, backed up by data, and it has some intuitive appeal ... Who hasn't wondered if they were single because they weren't pretty enough? And every well-meaning relative will tell us our "time is running out"!

What is less well publicized is that the same research (Buss, 1989; Buss et al., 1990) also found that women and men were more similar than different in what they looked for in a mate. Although women desired mates who have the ability to invest resources, and men desire mates who display cues to youth and physical attractiveness, *both* sexes across cultures showed preferences for traits such as kindness, understanding, intelligence, and health.

So, just be careful: A lot of the theories you'll find on dating and mating are, at worst, the personal viewpoint of the author, and, at best, backed loosely by some kind of data that may or may not have been accurately interpreted and reported. Finally, even the best "science" is based on statistical significance and samples, i.e. what is true for a majority of the people studied. And, unless you or your dates have been going around volunteering for a multitude of research studies, those people aren't you! Therefore, taking any data or any theory as unequivocally personally relevant to you can be highly problematic.

MY PERSPECTIVE ON THE "GOOD WIFE" THING

Because people are highly self-referential, everyone believes what they value is what everyone else values. As an extension of this, we all have a false assumption that there is one market, and value in that market is assigned based on a universal set of principles – ours! The truth is that what is very high value for one person is not what is valued by another. Just like your friend might pay an obscene amount for shoes, while you'd prefer to spend the money on a holiday.

We all have worth in our own ways and will be seen as worthwhile (and marriageable if that is what we want) by the people who share those values. For example, I asked a local Balinese man when I visited that country how he came to choose his wife. He told me that he fell in love with her when he saw what good offerings she created for their village temple.

So, although society might still imply that there is something "wrong" with women who are single, we know that there are many different "rights" and therefore, it is no fault of the individual who, by choice or circumstance, remains unmarried. Although it sounds like a platitude, we are all unique and worthwhile in our own special ways. And later, we'll talk about how to honor your own uniqueness and stay authentic while dating (rather than trying to "sell" yourself to get a guy to like you).

Additionally, my view is that having someone fall in love with you is as much about *how* you are, as it is *who* you are. There is a lot of contradictory data on the question, 'Do opposites attract?' because it depends on what you are talking about: Values? Personality traits?

Attachment styles? The easier and more useful question to answer is *how* do you attract? And, assuming you want to find a partner, how do you attract someone with whom you can have a healthy relationship? Thanks to researchers such as John and Julie Gottman, we've got the data we need to answer to that question for you later in the book.

DOING SINGLE WELL: VALUES SHOPPING CENTER EXERCISE (ADAPTED FROM LEJEUNE, 2007)

Instructions: You are going shopping at the Values Shopping Center. All of the experiences or qualities that you buy will become a part of your life. The ones you don't buy will be absent from your life. You can buy as many items as you like from any aisle, or none at all. However, you have exactly $100 to spend. Since the value of each item varies for everyone, all of the prices in the Values Shopping Center have been randomly assigned.

AISLE 1: LEISURE AND LEARNING	
Traveling and / or adventure	$6
Learning new things	$8
Enjoying a sport or physical activity	$5
Enjoying the outdoors and nature	$6
Enjoying art, music, or literature	$7
Having a hobby	$7

AISLE 2: FAMILY AND FRIENDS	
Close relationships with family	$9
Hanging out and having fun with friends	$8
Emotional intimacy and sharing	$7
Meeting new people	$6
Belonging to a group	$8
Being popular and admired by many	$9

AISLE 3: CAREER	
Making a lot of money	$9
Ambition, growth, and (good) challenge	$8
Being able to be creative	$7
Helping others or contributing to society	$6
Doing something with work / life balance or flexibility	$9
Having power and / or authority	$7

AISLE 4: SPIRITUAL AND COMMUNITY	
Having a spiritual belief system and practice	$8
Belonging to a spiritual, political, cultural, or charitable community	$7
Being politically aware and involved	$6
Caring about animals and the environment	$9
Caring about fairness and social justice	$7

AISLE 5: MIND–BODY CONNECTION	
Eating healthy foods	$6
Exercising regularly	$7
Emotional intelligence	$9
Self-esteem	$6
Relaxation, meditation, and managing stress well	$7

CHAPTER 2

DATING DEVELOPMENTS
IN RECENT TIMES

To understand the dating landscape and the experience of single women currently, it is important to understand how dating has changed over the last few generations. To my mind, three developments are most notable in terms of their impact on dating and female sexuality. These were:

1. The introduction of the contraceptive pill and ensuing sexual revolution

2. The women's liberation movement which saw more women get access to paid employment

3. The introduction of online dating

For a more thorough account of the history and influences on single women I highly recommend *All the Single Ladies* by Rebecca Traister.

Just five years after its introduction in 1960, the contraceptive pill became the most popular form of birth control in the USA. With over 6.5 million American women taking it, the pill was credited as the catalyst of the sexual revolution. Before its introduction, condoms were the primary form of contraception. However, the condoms of the time were expensive, thick, had poor sensitivity, and poor quality control – and as such they either weren't effective or weren't used. The relative availability and effectiveness of the pill brought about an increased acceptance of sex outside of marriage: For the first time in history, women who weren't overly religious could have sex without risking falling pregnant! Women could therefore date and have sex with more men and postpone marriage if they could financially afford to do so.

And with the women's liberation movement of the late 1960s and early 1970s more women could afford to do so! Reforms initiated in this era by "second wave feminists" saw the increase of women in the workforce. These reforms included: fair hiring practices, paid maternity leave, affordable child care, equal pay for men and women performing equal roles, and equal access to educational and employment opportunities for women. As a result, it became much more viable for women to study and gain careers, and women began to see their roles not just as wives and mothers.

Improvements in household labor-saving technology (fridges, vacuums, washing machines, etc.) after World War II also played an important role in freeing up women's time to enter the workforce (Greenwood, Seshadri & Yorukoglu, 2005). This same technology boom led to the increasing use of computers in the home and business. By 1995 the world wide web had been introduced. 1998 saw email became a normal part of life and the film *You've Got Mail* starring Meg Ryan and Tom Hanks normalized finding love over the internet. In 2000, eHarmony became the first online dating site, and by 2007, smart phones were introduced allowing daters to communicate on the go. From 2012, location-based dating apps like Tinder became popular, and dating became as "easy" as swiping left or right. And all that internet technology has brought us here – to the dating climate inhabited by today's sexually free, financially independent single women.

A PERSONAL HISTORY

In order to understand the impact of these developments on how women experience single life today, I'm going to describe the experience of the women in my own family, going back two generations.

My paternal grandmother, Beatrice, was born in 1906 in Queensland, Australia. She was the second eldest of six children. She was from a poor family; her father was a saddler (which was not a great occupation to have when cars were coming in!). She went to state schools and then managed to get a scholarship to a commercial high school, where she learned bookkeeping, typing, and secretarial work. This enabled her to get a job as a librarian after she finished her schooling.

Beatrice met my grandfather at a dance in 1927. She was the school friend of the daughter of the local sawmill's boss, for whom my grandfather worked. It is thought that she was a virgin when she married and had little experience with men as her family were not church-goers and didn't have the money to be part of the society that would have had "coming out" balls and similar occasions.

They married in 1928, when she was 22 years old and my grandfather was 27 years old. In those days, married women weren't allowed to work, so she kept her marriage a secret until she became pregnant with her first son (my uncle) in 1936. It is thought that the delay in pregnancy was due to the Great Depression (1929–1940) where 25 percent of men were unemployed and my grandfather was out of a job for at least some of the time.

My maternal grandmother, Mercia, was born in 1914 in Sydney, Australia. She was the eldest of eight. Her father had emigrated to Australia from Lebanon when he was 10 years old, her mother had been born in Australia. They were Catholic and middle class – her father owned a general goods store.

At 27 years old, she was still unmarried and training to be a nurse, living in the nurses' quarters, when she met my grandfather at a dance held for young Lebanese singles in 1941. She was considered an old maid to be single at that age! Apparently, she had had a serious relationship with another man before this, which, for unknown reasons, didn't lead to marriage. She had wanted to finish her training but was never able to sit her final exams as my grandfather wouldn't wait to marry her, and married women were still not allowed to work. Three years later, she had her first of seven children. She never worked as a nurse but with two sets of twins she certainly had her work cut out!

My mother was the third of those seven children. She was born in 1950 in Sydney and her family were well-off financially. My grandfather had become successful through opening a chain of menswear stores. When my mother was 21 years old, she left home under a great deal of opposition from her family – it was still considered scandalous! She had trained in graphic design, and had begun working as an activities coordinator in an old age home, when she met my father in 1976. She met him at a party where he had been the date of one of her girlfriends. She was married to him six months later at 26 years old, and I was born five years after this. She was going to university to study to be a psychologist while she was pregnant with me, and was able to work throughout my childhood in her own business.

Mum says she had lots of boyfriends, and lots of sex before she was married. She said that she first got the contraceptive pill in her early twenties, but would never have told her very Catholic parents about that! My mother says that my father was the first man she introduced to the family and that there was a lot of pressure for her to marry him when she did so. Because of the contraceptive pill I was one of only three children. Mum said she had my sister three years later to be a playmate for me, and my baby sister – 13 years my junior – was a happy surprise.

I still remember my mother typing out her university assignments on her typewriter. Our family got our first Commodore 64 computer when I was about eight years old, in 1989. In high school we would call friends on their house landlines after school, only switching to internet messaging in my final year of high school (1998). I remember having an old Nokia phone and only upgrading to a fancy new iPhone with internet capability when I was 27 years old, in 2008.

My first few boyfriends were boys I had met at parties in high school and university. I had gone on the contraceptive pill when I was 18 years old. My parents were very open minded; they were happy for me to have sex as long as I didn't get pregnant. I remember having my boyfriends sleep over in my room while I was living at home.

It wasn't until the end of my seven-year (and only de facto) relationship in 2008 that I got my first taste of internet dating. I hated it! At the time there were only boring, long-winded computer-based programs available like eHarmony and RSVP. All that reading and emailing! Speed dating was fun but generally unproductive. Meeting new men generally happened at bars while I was out with friends ... until one by one, my friends got married and stopped going out so much. Then came Tinder ...

As you can see, no previous generation of women has had the experience that the current generation is having. Only two generations ago, the lifestyles and expectations for women were unrecognizably different. Even in my own twenties, internet dating was considered rare (and for losers). Social change takes time and social attitudes can linger long after changes have taken place. Is it any wonder that we still get older relatives at weddings telling us "our time is running out" and warning us that "all the good ones will be taken"?

DOING SINGLE WELL: YOUR OWN STORY

Interview your parents and family members about their dating experiences and the expectations on them as they grew up. Ask them about your grandparents if they aren't around to ask yourself. Ask about careers, dating, sex. Where did they meet people? How old were they when they married? Did they experience any pressure to conform to societal norms at the time? See if you can build a picture of what life was like for women in your mother and grandmother's era and culture. Then compare that to your own story. How might someone from your mother's era view your life now? What about someone from your grandmother's era?

Feel free to post what you find out on our Facebook page @doingsinglewell

CHAPTER 3

THE PLEASURES AND PITFALLS OF MODERN DATING

The opportunities available to women have undoubtedly improved over recent generations. However, more choice and more possibilities can have a surprisingly negative effect: with choice and freedom comes ambiguity, uncertainty, and stress. Although women *are* more liberated, there are certain aspects of that liberation which can be seen to make dating more difficult than it was before.

RELATIONSHIP ROULETTE

Back in our grandparents' days things could be seen to have been relatively simple. A woman would choose the most appropriate marital partner in her limited social circle when she was at the appropriate age. The world was a much smaller place, without everyone having their own car, and without easily available international travel. Communities were closer, choices were more simple, and the internet was decades away.

There was also far less ambiguity in dating: if a man was interested in you, he would court you in the usual way, and you could assume his intentions were marriage. A "rogue and a scoundrel" was easy to spot for being inappropriate and *not* following this script. Nowadays, what is appropriate is up to the individual. There is a veritable smorgasbord of relationship models to choose from. So whether we are hungry for a hook-up, craving casual sex, whether we want a same-sex friend-with-benefits, or prefer polyamory, almost any dating delicacy can be made to order. The difficulty then comes with working out what we want, and finding someone who wants the same!

Having increased opportunity and more options doesn't mean people necessarily know what type of relationship they want when they begin dating – they may even use the dating process as a means of working it out. Moreover, what someone wants can also change depending on *who* it's with. "It's complicated" is becoming an increasingly common relationship status and "it depends!" is no longer necessarily an evasive response if you ask a date what he's looking for.

We would never be expected to accept a job with a company that doesn't really know what our job description is, but increasingly women (and men) are accepting this level of ambiguity as a normal part of modern dating.

'I once went out with a guy for three months when, one night over margaritas, he tells me that he is really enjoying me being "one of his partners" and would I be interested in meeting his "other friend"? ... Here I was thinking about asking if he wanted to meet my parents!' – Jill, 29 years old.

THE LIBERATION PARADOX

Good communication is vital to navigating the ambiguity of modern dating with our sanity intact! However, communicating what we want, and exploring what our date is in the market for, can be an awkward set of conversations for the less assertive. I often find one of the difficulties single women have is being upfront about what they want, particularly if what they want is marriage and babies. Although society still pushes us to want these things, there now seems to be a certain amount of shame about wanting them, and a belief that by declaring it, we are at risk of scaring off a date.

Sally Cline (1994) and Naomi Wolf (1997) wrote of the paradox that the sexual liberation was actually *male* liberation! The pill removed a justifiable excuse for women to refuse unwanted sexual advances, gave men more access to women's bodies, and justified male promiscuity. Whether or not you hold this to be true, there does seem to be a dominant discourse in today's society that men want sex, and asking for commitment can scare them off.

However, there is also an idea that if we give men sex "too easily," they won't respect us and see us as good wife material. This "Madonna-whore complex," first coined by Freud in 1912, is one of many paradoxes for single women as a consequence of increased choices and opportunity. As modern women we have to like sex and be sexually liberated, but we can't give it away too easily or with too many partners, or men won't respect us and want to marry us.

It is these double-binds or mixed messages in today's society that can leave women confused, anxious, and unable to ask for what they want when dating. As such, it seems that modern women have more options. But in truth there are still social norms and society scripts that men and women are supposed to follow, that just make things more complicated!

'I don't know what men want anymore. I met a guy on Tinder and we hooked up. I liked him and the sex was good so we struck up a more regular physical thing. Then, out-of-the-blue he starts getting all preachy on me! Asking me who else I was sleeping with, and telling me I had low self-esteem, and I shouldn't be giving myself away so easily ... ummm pot-kettle much?!' – Kellie, 35 years old.

THE DIFFICULTIES OF DELAY

The modern postponement of forming committed relationships often means, for better and for worse, that we are more likely to know who we are by the time we meet our life partners. Postponing settling down until our late twenties and thirties means that we are no longer malleable teenagers and have a more defined, possibly inflexible, sense of self. The more sophisticated our self-concept becomes, the harder it can be for us to accept someone who is not a great fit for us. How many of us would still choose our high-school sweethearts? Ironically, the greater variation we are afforded in gender role preference, and the more varied our life experience has been, the more difficult it can be to find someone who is well suited to us.

Delay of marriage in the service of education, self-development, travel, and career has also brought about the common problem single women have of "racing their biological clock." Today we are told that we can and should have it all (meaning a career, and marriage, and family) but just as there is still a glass ceiling for women in terms of career advancement, there is still a biological road block where a woman's fertility declines as she gets older. The Western cultural shift towards later pregnancy has spurred the rapid advancement in reproductive technology. However, the experience of most single women who want children is one of stress and pressure, feeling pushed for time to secure their futures, both in career and family life.

'I've always loved travel and so when I got a job that meant I'd get to travel all over the world I was delighted! I met a ton of people and had the most amazing experiences, but I got tired and decided it was about time to come home and settle down (much to my family's delight!). The only problem is I don't fit in anymore. All my high-school girlfriends are married with kids and the people I meet are so insular, I don't feel we have a lot in common. My friend pointed out that I tend to date guys who are here on working visas – and I do! They are my people! But not good marriage material!' – Mia, 36 years old.

"PICKING" PROBLEMS

Entering academic life and the workforce has given women the ability to access a broader dating pool. With the advent of internet dating, that pool has become almost limitless, and dating can occur with minimal effort – the click of a few buttons or the swipe of a finger. Yet, even this is a double-edged sword. Who do you choose if your choices are limitless? Does having limitless choice really help you meet good relationship candidates, or do you just waste more time on people whom you would never have met in your real life, and who aren't similar enough to you to be good candidates?

In my experience, the more dates a woman goes on where there is little connection, the more discouraged and dispirited she can become about the whole dating process. To prevent running out of steam it would be easy to assume that being more selective is the way to go. However, the reverse is also true: the relative de-personalization that has occurred with the rise of internet dating means that women can also err on the side of being too picky online!

If you met a guy at a bar or at a party, politeness would give you the opportunity for the type of human connection that might help you look past superficial first impressions. Then, if there was enough of a connection, you may be willing to forgive the fact that the man you were speaking with wasn't *exactly* right. For example, you might overlook that he doesn't have a post-graduate degree if you felt strongly enough for him, even if you had always thought post-graduate qualifications were important.

The internet dating phenomenon has resulted in people using different, and perhaps more unforgiving selection criteria on which to base their dating judgments. On the internet we get a surplus of (dubiously accurate) information *before* we even begin to interact. We can get caught in their checklists of what makes a good match and can lean towards making false negative errors: Screening out good dates because they don't fit our ideal criteria or aren't attractive enough in their photos.

Here's a story of one of my clients to show you what I mean let's call her Ms T (for Tinderiffic):

Ms T arrived for her appointment one Monday in a flap. She was agitated and literally wringing her hands. When I asked her what was up, she looked at me bashfully and explained that she had been to the races on the weekend, and one of her married-with-babies girlfriends had gotten her phone and blithely taken over her Tinder account. Ms T had not previously had much success finding anyone to date, but woke up on Sunday to a ton of text messages, and a reminder that she had "agreed" to go on a date that week!

Now although I don't condone identity theft generally, I asked to see her phone and the people she had been matched with. I saw their pictures and read the initial message exchanges. They all looked like perfectly normal, polite guys to me! I asked her what she imagined the problem would be if she went on the date. She looked at me in horror and said, 'but he's wearing a hat!' I looked at the photo again, just a regular guy in a baseball cap ... 'He could be bald!' she explained ...

I handed the phone back to her and asked her to pick three features from his photos that she liked. She said she liked his green eyes, he had a nice smile and she liked that his photo was taken on the beach, because she also liked the beach. I then asked her to read out loud the message exchange between him and her girlfriend. She agreed he was polite, seemed open and genuine, had asked questions about her (or her girlfriend at least) and had made a couple of good jokes. I then asked her again what the problem would be if she went on a date with him ...

Lo and behold, Ms T went on her date and came back to me the following week with a smile. They had had a picnic and taken a sunset walk along the beach followed by a twilight dip in the ocean pool. The date had lasted four hours, and she had found him relaxed and entertaining. He was balding but far from that being a turn-off, she told me that his lack of perfection had made her feel more comfortable stripping down to her bikini on the first date.

The moral of this story is that looks don't matter a great deal when there is a good connection, so I urge you to be generous when internet dating. Liking someone on an app is not promising to marry them, so you can afford to be a little left-swiping trigger happy. I generally recommend saying "yes" to anyone who looks like he would fit in at a dinner or at the pub with your friends ... you can always filter them out later on!

LAZY DATERS

'It's like online job applications, you can target many people simultaneously and hope that one of them will stick.' – Emily, 26 years old.

Limitless choices can make people both picky and lazy! Because there are so many candidates, both male and female daters can put a lot less effort into getting to know someone. Faced with a never-ending stream of singles online, and the lack of face-to-face repercussions for rudeness, daters can connect with a multitude of singles simultaneously and then drop out of contact just as easily. There is little need for charm and social graces and a lot of "dating" ends abruptly before any face-to-face contact has been made.

Traditional courtship – picking up the telephone and asking someone on a date – required courage, planning, and resilience. Not so with "asynchronous communication" like texting and email, where you can ask a question and not get a reply straightaway. Daters don't invest much time, money, or care and with such a complacent attitude, dating loses its sense of excitement and fun. The likelihood of finding a connection can decrease.

Laziness can come in other forms too: People who were previously too shy to approach a potential date in a bar or social situation are able to find false confidence behind the safety of a screen. Internet technology has created a convenient way for people to avoid the painful anxieties of meeting new people and being vulnerable. It is one thing to send an (overly edited and vetted-by-a-friend) text message. It's a completely different and more challenging prospect to sit opposite someone, just the two of you, and discuss your real thoughts on an issue, to share yourself and your reactions in real time.

Similarly, people who were too busy to date can now pretend to have the time via late-night online chat from the comfort of their couches. The ease of modern technology makes it possible to chat online or via SMS for weeks before actually meeting a person on a real date! But can you really count yourself as available and see yourself as dating if you only really have the time or confidence for some late-night swiping? Are armchair-daters really ready and committed to put in the effort it takes to form a relationship that will last through good times and bad?

To show you what I mean here is the story of one of my clients, let's call her Ms V (for Very Busy).

Ms V came to me because she had made a New Year's resolution to find a partner. She hadn't been in a serious relationship for more than seven years. Most of her recent experiences with men had been overseas hook-ups while on work trips, and an ongoing, long-distance internet-based flirtation with a work colleague in another country. I gave her my lecture on unavailable men (see Chapter 12). Then, because she was open to internet dating (she'd tried it a few times before) I got her to download some apps and create her profile. The following week she was doing well, she had five people she was chatting to, she'd filtered out the inappropriate ones, and she said she was having fun. She cancelled her next appointment and I thought, 'Fantastic! She's met someone!'

Two months later she walked through my door again. I asked her how it had gone, and she looked at me blankly. I reminded her of the five guys she had been chatting to and she laughed and said, 'Oh you know, they all fizzled out like they always do!' I asked to see the messages ... sure enough, in all five cases the texts had fizzled. However, it seemed *she* was the culprit. One guy had asked to meet her for a drink and she'd not responded for four days. Another had suggested that they meet up and she'd said she was busy, and given him a date two weeks away. When I asked her about this she said that her work had been very busy and she'd been called overseas on a couple of occasions which had meant she hadn't had much free time.

I asked her to think back to a time she might have had a different goal: losing weight, learning a language, or an instrument. I asked her to imagine how far she would get with her goal if she only ever went to the gym or picked up her French book or guitar once every two weeks. She could see that this wasn't enough of a commitment to get her anywhere. I then asked her to imagine that she had a live-in partner already ... How often would she have spent quality time with him recently? She cringed and admitted she hadn't been home before 9pm any night that week.

Ms V agreed that in fact she was unavailable. We explored her history and attitudes to help her understand why she had been working so hard, and why she had been putting herself (and her personal life) on the back burner. I'm pleased to say that she has since switched companies and now has a role involving far less travel. She now has a dog *and* a partner!

ROBO-CONNECTION

SMS, email, Instagram, Facebook, and Snapchat (to name a few) have fundamentally changed our communication habits, and continue to pose large challenges to our human attachment and bonding processes.

With text-based communication we miss out on the all-important cues of tone of voice, inflection, and body language. This introduces many ambiguities that can become a hotbed for anxiety and obsessional thinking. Who hasn't agonized over what an ambiguous text or WhatsApp message means? Moreover, in case we didn't get our fill the first time, text-based communication can be stored for later retrieval, re-reading and endless out-of-context over-analysis – what fun!

Text-based communications are asynchronous – which just means we don't know when the recipient will get our message. As anyone who has been on the receiving end of an unanswered text knows, the delay can really increase our anxiety and insecurity. And that can interfere with forming a secure attachment. Similarly, if we delay texting to consult a friend, to perfect our next text message, or just so we can play it cool, it means we're bastardizing the bonding process. Whoever we're communicating with is not getting the real deal!

'When I met my boyfriend's best friend I knew something was up. The chick was weird and couldn't look me in the eyes. At first, I thought something had happened between them, but it turns out she was embarrassed because she was the one who had originally been replying to my texts for him! I'm still not sure how I feel about that!' – Lisa, 34 years old.

With more and more information about everyone publicly available, and more beautiful people to compare ourselves to, we are all feeling a lot less worthy, and a lot more insecure. Social media and image-editing technology put greater pressure on us to fit in, play it cool, be liked or followed – and to be perfect. Our relationships are becoming more screen–based, less intimate, and less real. For what is a close friend but someone who knows and loves us warts and all? Can we call someone our bestie if we can't count on them to be there, in person, on our couch, eating ice cream with us on the lonely nights?

Achieving self-esteem and intimacy will never happen when we try to fit in and be liked. True connection can only happen when we are brave enough to be ourselves in all our perfect imperfection. The robo-connection of modern technology will never be an adequate substitute for eye-to-eye, face-to-face, real-time, real-you sharing.

DOING SINGLE WELL: MINDFULNESS OF SOCIAL MEDIA

Have you ever stopped to think about how social media affects you? How often do you check it? Why? How does it leave you feeling?

Mindfulness can help. This is a process whereby you take an "observer" position with yourself and watch your own process as it happens. That means paying attention to your thoughts, feelings, body sensations, and action urges before, during, and after you next check your social media.

What do you notice about your patterns? Are there certain feelings or thoughts that provoke you to check social media? Are there certain posts which make you feel good or bad? Do you feel better or worse about yourself after checking it? Put your thoughts down here:

QUICK TIPS ON TECHNO DATING

– Be generous in your selection criteria on internet dating sites, and meet your dates ASAP. You never know how well you'll click until you meet them face-to-face.

– Keep the text-based communication to a minimum. Pick up the phone! I tell my clients that unless you're texting an address, it is probably better said than written.

– Meaningful connections require effort and vulnerability. If you are not willing to be anxious, put in the time and money or "show up" authentically, then you might need to ask yourself if you really want to be in a relationship.

– If there is any ambiguity, ask about it. 'You haven't called when you said you would, does this mean you aren't really interested in pursuing this?'

At best, this will clarify the situation. At worst, it will confirm your interpretation. This may seem uncool, but as you will read as we work through the book, authenticity is more likely to be attractive and lead you to successful connections than being cool ever will!

A RISE IN RUDENESS

The depersonalization of internet dating can also give rise to online bullying, unwanted sexual photos and texts, and general meanness that would rarely occur with face-to-face meetings and telephone conversations. Being able to send a nasty or lewd text, safe in the knowledge that your date doesn't know you, and won't be able to do anything about it, is the dark side of the advances in dating technology.

What about "ghosting" and "bread crumbing"? Not responding to a date, or continuing to feed them tiny morsels of contact rather then tell them you're not interested, is both a blessing, to those who find rejecting someone difficult, and a curse to those who would prefer to be told upfront. Similarly, having any number of willing sexual partners on hand at the click of a button can be a boon for the sexually liberated woman, but can also lead to a greater risk of sexual assault and sexually transmitted disease for those who judge poorly. And yes, that could actually be any one of us, because what can we really tell about a person from a couple of photos and some texts?!

'There is nothing gentlemanly about internet dating! The amount of dick pics I've been sent I could put together a coffee-table book! I just don't get how guys think that's a turn-on?!' – Rae, 26 years old.

THE PROBLEM OF PORN

Last but not at all least, high-speed internet has also given rise to readily available pornography. Pornography generally portrays a certain type of sex, a "masculine" sexuality, where sexual variety, sexy costumes, toys, group sex, orgasms and cum shots reign supreme. People in pornos have very specific body types and a very specific type of unemotional sex.

There is a great deal of research being done on the effect of this on our sexuality. From my perspective, it gives rise to a highly transactional form of sex that is easy to obtain via the dating apps, but not very fulfilling for either gender. So where are the alternative models? When was the last time you got to witness a loving and emotionally connected sexual encounter?

What will happen in our relationships when we become so used to sexual novelty and plastic bodies through pornography that we can't get turned on by our familiar, natural-bodied partners? Although porn addiction – an ever-growing compulsion to view pornographic material – is a huge problem, I'm just as concerned about the "normal" porn user. The perception now seems to be that it is considered normal to have viewed, or even regularly view, some kind of porn. Modern dieticians are demonizing sugar and processed foods, saying that although these things have been considered a normal part of our diet, they are actually quite bad for us. Similarly, I think the normalization of porn has an equal, if not greater, widespread toxic impact.

'The last guy I took home asked me if I could squirt for him ... after he left I had to look up what he meant!' – Zoe, 23 years old.

PART II

SINGLE WOMAN, "KNOW THYSELF!"

We don't need it to be written on the walls or told to us by some ancient Greek dudes in sheets to know that knowing ourselves is going to be of huge benefit when it comes to living the best life we can. As such, the starting point in being able to "Do Single Well" is looking at our internal world and getting to know ourselves: what thoughts, feelings, and choices are causing us to feel more "desperate and dateless" than "satisfied single woman"?

This section details the most common unhelpful thoughts we can have, including myths about men and our own "gremlins" (unhelpful beliefs about ourselves). It will give practical strategies for managing these thoughts. We will be challenged to change our view on what is attractive, and encouraged to try a new recipe for becoming our most attractive selves. We will also delve into the common uncomfortable feelings that come up for single women and how to best manage them. Finally, we will explore avoidance, so we can work out if we are really putting our best foot forward as a single woman or just finding excuses to stay in our current situation.

CHAPTER 4

MYTHS ABOUT MEN AND WHY WE BELIEVE THEM

One of the first things to check ourselves for is a case of the man myths! Like bad pick-up lines, a man myth is easy to spot for its familiar, but unenticing, reek of cliché, resignation, and hopelessness. Always over-generalized, never helpful, these myths become the mantra of defeat that give some women justification for why they're still single.

To try to debunk these myths, I sought out population data and scientific research to help convince my single women that men weren't as dastardly as they had found themselves believing. I was soon to learn that despite my very nerdy and conscientious approach, people rarely let facts get in the way of a good bias! No matter how many facts I presented, if someone was determined to blame the boys, she would. Like an old tatty blanket that is clung to for safety in the big wide world of dating, some ladies were so resistant to giving up their much-loved man myths they would even take it as a personal challenge to google opposing data and disprove me!

So, dear single women, instead of providing you with statistics and data, which will likely be outdated by the time you read this, I'm going to take a different approach: I'm going to name the man myths that you may have heard, or even spread yourself. I'm going to tell you why it is unhelpful to think like this, whether you think there is any truth to these myths or not. And I'm going to offer an explanation for why it's so appealing to trot out this rot every time you feel discouraged.

MYTH 1: ALL THE GOOD ONES ARE TAKEN

'It's such slim pickings out there. My friends have found lovely partners, but it seems all the good ones are taken, and I'd rather be alone than have to settle for some of the guys I meet.' – Jean, 34 years old.

It is so easy to get discouraged and to think that because we've had a run of bad dates there are no decent, available guys left. Perhaps you even use this reasoning to talk yourself out of putting effort into dating? Of course, when we're thinking like this, we will conveniently forget about the ample evidence that "bad ones" are taken too. We'll forget how over martinis last week, our best friend complained about the numerous failings of her husband; or the story on Facebook about the guy who was two-timing his pregnant-with-twins wife ...

To the disenchanted single mind, the men in a relationship are the "good ones" and those that are left are "bad"!

Yet, we all know that both good people and bad people can fall on hard times, and have bad things happen to them. That means that both good and bad people (let's call them "relationship-ready" and "unsuitables") will have various life events that cause them to be single at various times. Whether it be due to a mismatched first marriage, being the victim of an affair, being a shy guy, being a widower, or being someone who has had other focuses in life, there are plenty of reasons a guy might be single that do not put him in the "unsuitable" category.

Of course, past-relationship history is an important topic to explore when dating a new person. It is true that men who are unsuitable can be single because they have had many failed relationships, or a relative lack of relationships in their history. It is also true that we need to be very wary of a guy who blames his ex-partner or his circumstances for his current single status in a "victim" type of way. Relationships are two-way streets and any guy who can't take responsibility for his part in previous relationship failure should be given a wide berth. However, this is by no means the majority of men, and so to make the sweeping binary classification "that all the good ones are taken" will lead us to making a false negative error: We will overlook all the very good relationship-ready men out there!

Men (and women!) can be unsuitable for a relationship because of their poor relationship skills and attitudes. Or, temporary circumstances might make them unavailable for a relationship at a particular time. Sure, no matter which type of "unsuitable" man you've been burned by in the past, it still hurts! But it would be a mistake to assume that all the guys with whom it didn't work out were "bad" guys.

Whether you've met them or not, there are heaps of guys who are relationship-ready, and if you can let go of this bitter belief that "all the good ones are taken," you can become relationship-ready too!

DOING SINGLE WELL: CIRCUMSTANCES CHANGE

Still not convinced? Think about all the people you know who have been single at some time in their adult lives. Were they all unsuitable? Have none of them gone on to have happy relationships? Would you like someone to assume you are unsuitable just because you're currently single? Have a go at journaling your thoughts below and post your stories on Facebook @doingsinglewell

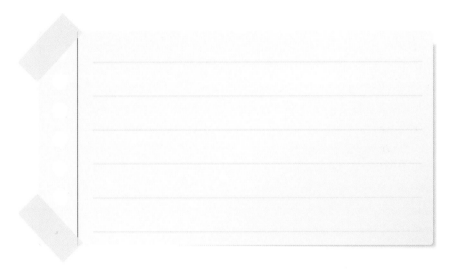

To illustrate this point I'm going to tell you about my client, let's call her Ms S (for Second Chance):

Ms S came to me to discuss a dating opportunity she had. She had not been in a relationship for many years as she had been busy pursuing a very intense career in a national sporting team. She'd hooked up with fellow sportsmen, but the touring schedule was rough on relationships, and in that industry, everyone had to put their career and their teams first. In fact, the only relationship she'd been in was with a high-school sweetheart who'd broken her heart when he moved overseas to pursue his career. Because they had mutual friends she found out that he'd been something of a player overseas at first. Hers had not been the only heart left in tatters!

Despite this, they had reconnected at a wedding a year ago, and had been in friendly email contact since. He was in a relationship and she hadn't thought much of the casual contact until she received an email saying that he was moving back to Sydney, without his now ex-partner and wanted to take her on a date. She was excited, but anxious. On the one hand he was a smart, sensitive guy who had made a good name for himself in his career, and had said he wanted to settle down and have kids. On the other hand, he'd put his career first, been a player, and hadn't been committed to his last partner ... To be single at 35 ... surely there must be something wrong with him?!

I spoke with her about how he'd described his recent break-up – he'd told her that it was an amicable one; they had just grown apart. In the end, he had wanted to move back, to be near his family, and start one of his own, but she hadn't wanted to do that. I asked Ms S if there was any reason, apart from their history – now 10 years in the past – and her own singlism that made her believe he was "unsuitable." She said no. Then, you guessed it, I told her to go on the date. One date led to more and within six months Ms S was in my office with Mr. S in tow! He had asked her to marry him and she was back for pre-marital counseling to make sure they gave their marriage the best chance they could!

MYTH 2: ALL MEN ARE PLAYERS

'I've never been internet dating – all those guys online are only after one thing. I'm more traditional, I'm not into hook-ups ... but guys will be guys nowadays. Chivalry is dead, and it feels like because of this I'll be single forever!' – Sally, 36 years old.

I feel a bit sorry for men these days. On the one hand, they are given the constant messaging that to be a "real man" they have to think about sex, want sex, be good at sex, pursue sex, and be up for sex whenever it's offered. And we women are not at all faultless in perpetuating the pressure! Although we will often talk about men being players in a disparaging way, truthfully speaking, what would you think of a man who didn't try to make any moves on you at all after the first few dates?!

On the other hand, these same men are also told to respect women, that their sex drive is shameful and causes rape, and that their sexual fantasies are dirty and demeaning to women. 'Be a "real man" but not a pervert,' 'Pursue but don't ever be pushy,' 'Be sexually proficient but not a player,' 'Have desire but don't be a dick about it.' Men are in such a double-bind that it's a wonder there are any still brave enough to even try their hand at dating!

If we took it as a biological truth that higher testosterone levels result in higher libido then, yes, most men will have a higher libido than most women. However, biology does not solely determine behavior and, just like with women, there are many factors including stress; performance anxiety; body image issues; physical health and fitness; and lack of emotional connection, which mean that the men we meet may *not* always be gagging for it.

It is also true that a lot of men have been socialized to express themselves physically rather than through the more "feminine" channels of talking. As Cher sang, 'If you wanna know if he loves you so, it's in his kiss.' Indeed, I have seen many men who get plenty of sex, but end up feeling empty and unfulfilled in their relationships or hook-ups. These men actually want love and connection, but have never been taught any socially acceptable "masculine" way to access it, other than via sex.

However, just as little girls *and* little boys love and need the love of their caregivers equally, so grown-up women *and* grown-up men love and desire the love of their partners equally. We *all* want to love and be loved. Both genders seek relationships where they can be seen, heard, and understood.

Often men feel least understood when it comes to their libido. From 'Don't touch that or you'll go blind' to 'Not again, you are such an animal!' men are taught to feel bad about their sex drives from boyhood into adulthood. This shaming can have negative effects on how a man expresses himself sexually. For example, a normal defense mechanism against shame is to project that shame onto their partners. It may be easier for him to feel that she is wrong, or deficient in some way, and be angry at her for not wanting sex, or wanting more than just sex, than it is to feel bad things about himself!

I'm not excusing a man who pushes a woman for sex, can't take no for an answer, acts like a sex pest, or complains about a woman's lack of sex drive. In fact, I advise all single women who experience this to set very clear, firm boundaries and walk away immediately if those boundaries are not respected! However, I am saying that if we looked a little deeper into the drivers for these behaviors in men, we might find that they aren't all as dastardly as we make them out to be. They are often just as confused, just as needy for love and compassion, and just as lost as we are.

Yes, you may well meet men who are players: who only want casual sex, and are therefore unsuitable for dating, unless you just want casual sex too. But these men are easy to spot. Casual sex is so permissible these days that few men feel the need to mislead women into thinking they want a relationship, when all they really want is sex! They'll write it in their profiles, their chat will quickly turn sexual, they'll ask you to come to their place, or go to yours for a first date; they may even send you a dick pic! It couldn't really be clearer!

Your role as a single woman is to not be one of those ladies who try to barter sex for love. I've so often heard women say that they thought that if they shared a good enough sexual connection with a guy, he would eventually fall in love and want more. However, good sex rarely makes someone relationship-ready, so why waste your time on the gamble when there are plenty of relationship-ready men out there?

In the end, if all men wanted was sex, and all men were in fact players, there would not be so many married, family-oriented men around. Our society structure as a whole would have gone through far greater revolution than it has. In this era where marriage is optional, divorce is easy, and hook-up platforms abound, it would be very easy for players to keep playing until their hearts were content. Yet, this is not really the world we are living in.

In real life, both men and women tend to give up counting the notches on their bedposts, and eventually want to settle down. So, if you would like to consider yourself relationship-ready, you would be better off: reflecting on your attitudes about men and sex; ensuring you feel confident saying 'no' if you need to; screening out whatever players you do come across; and dating the remaining men with a sense of compassion for the tough role they have to play in this dating caper.

To illustrate my point I'll tell you a story about one of my clients, let's call him Mr. I (for Intimacy):

Mr. I came to me shortly after his 27th birthday. He had broken up from his first and only long-term relationship six months previously, and had begun dating again. He looked embarrassed as he admitted that it wasn't as much fun as he had imagined it would be, and he didn't think he had any "game."

When I asked him what he meant, he said that a lot of his friends were envious of him being single, but that he felt he wasn't suited to dating. He'd been on a number of dates with nice girls, but he felt he wasn't meeting their expectations as he didn't want to kiss them. 'What never?!' I asked … He said no, of course not "never," but rarely in the first few dates. He said he liked to get to know someone before becoming sexual, but he'd felt pressure from the girls he was dating.

One girl had jumped on him in the car after their second date and, when he'd extracted himself and tried to explain, she'd stormed off and called him gay. He'd been on a handful of dates with the next one before she texted him and told him that she didn't think they had any "spark" (he'd kissed her goodbye, but they hadn't really gotten to trying anything else). By the time the last girl he'd dated had come along he'd been desperate to try something different and asked her to come home with him. They'd been fooling around and having fun, but he was nervous and his penis wasn't coming to the party. He'd assured her that he was interested in seeing her again, but she left that night and he'd never heard from her again. He'd never had problems with impotence before, but he felt hopeless – like he wasn't a "real man."

I assured him that it was totally okay for him to want to have some emotional intimacy before getting sexual, just as it was totally okay if someone wanted to have a casual hook-up. The key, I explained, was being honest about what you were into, and finding someone who was into the same thing. We spoke about how, and when, he could raise the issue, what he could say to satisfy someone who became insecure that she wasn't hot enough, or felt like he wasn't into her, and how to take rejection from anyone who was wanting something else.

Of course, once his confidence grew and he gave himself permission to want what he wanted, he found it easier to deal with rejection and eventually found a lovely lady who was more than happy to be wooed his way.

DOING SINGLE WELL: MAN–UP!

Put the shoe on the other foot. Imagine the gender roles have been reversed and it is now normal, if not obligatory, for women to make the first move sexually, and be the sexual pursuers in any relationship. How would you express your desire for sex? When would you? What would you feel and do if your overture was rejected? What would you do if you didn't feel like having sex but were expected to want it? Feel free to comment on @doingsinglewell

MYTH 3: ALL MEN WANT YOUNGER WOMEN

'I wish I'd started earlier. All the men at my age are looking for girls 20 years their junior, and it's such slim pickings among men out there that they can get them too!' – Sue, 65 years old.

The myth that all men want younger women is one of the trickiest to move beyond. Like all beliefs, when there is *some* truth to them, it's easy to overgeneralize and hold them to be true always. Although the pattern is slowly changing, it is true that it's more common for a man to be with a younger woman, than for a woman to be with a younger man.

However, it's also true that the majority of people will be with someone of a near or equivalent age to them. To see what is true for the age norms in your own community, have a think about the ages of your friends and colleagues compared to their partners.

There are many reasons why the stereotype that men desire younger women might be held. Youth is synonymous with beauty, and in this superficial, beauty-driven culture that we live in, we can all get seduced into finding youth attractive. Younger women may also have more chance of being able to have babies unassisted, which might be the reason for a family-oriented man to choose a younger woman. Yet, although I'm sure that there have been a number of men that have chosen significantly younger partners for these reasons among others, these men are not *all* men.

So, instead of giving up and feeling over the hill, if you consider yourself to be an older woman, take heart! Just have a think about the type of men who would value the beauty of youth ... are these really the kind of men you want?! If your answer is yes, you may have some work to do in healing your own ageism and body image shame. Youth is just one *type* of beauty. Think about all the extremely beautiful older women in the media now – could you really say that Glenn Close or Helen Mirren aren't magnificent? If you don't feel beautiful or desirable as an older woman, then it is certainly time to explore why, and do whatever you need to do to reclaim a healthy body image and self-esteem.

THE MIRACLE ANTI-AGEISM FORMULA:

- Make sure you are not around people who are ageist towards themselves or others. They'll be easy to pick for their complaints about wrinkles and getting older!

- Notice your own internal dialogue about your body and your age – try to call the lines on your face "storylines" rather than "wrinkles" and try to view your body as just as worthy of care and kindness as that of a baby (babies are often also kind of wrinkly, rolly, and funny looking too if you think about it!).

- Never continue to date someone who makes derogatory comments about your body or your age. There will always be haters, but we get to choose who to surround ourselves with, and we need to choose people who can love us for who we are.

- Make sure you are prioritizing your self-care and not letting yourself "go to seed" because of some unhelpful notion that "no one is looking anyway."

- Buy the clothes you like, even if you feel like "mutton dressed up as lamb" and stop covering your body in your dark-colored muumuus of shame. Celebrate the body you are in, and dress in whatever way makes you feel visible and good! If you need inspiration, then the work of photographer Ari Seth Cohen who produced the book Advanced Style is a great place to start.

- Begin making eye contact and smiling at people (especially men!) when you go out. A lot of my older single women complain that people stopped looking at them when they hit 40. I would counter-propose that they stopped looking for people who were looking when they began to feel ashamed of their age!

- And of course, if this is a bigger issue in your life than these strategies adequately address, do get the help of a body image therapist. You are worth whatever it takes to feel good about yourself.

For those of you who feel passed over for baby-making, I do understand that not being able to have a family when you want one can be one of the most painful situations someone can endure. In the next chapter, I'll share some helpful tips on how to deal with the issue of the dreaded biological clock.

The good news is that there are plenty of men who value the life experience and similar-mindedness of a same-age partner at any age. The excellent news is that you only need to find one of those men. So, no matter how many men you hear of who have chosen younger women, there will always be those that don't.

Here is an example from one of my clients, let's call her Ms F (for Fabulously Forty):

Ms F sat down for our first session and promptly burst into tears. She had met a man and fallen in love with him, and now she had to break up with him. 'Why?!' I asked. It turns out Ms F had decided she needed to end it because of their age gap.

They had met at a local café in passing, he had seen her and gotten the café owner to pass on his number when she next came in. They'd dated and found that they had a lot in common. She even said that his energy for life made her feel young again.

Despite the warnings of her friends ('He's on the rebound,' 'He just wants a visa,' 'He's playing you') they had such a good time together that neither of them wanted to end it. However, his age (29) had been eating away at her, and by the time she came to see me, she was convinced that she would get dumped for a "younger model."

I asked her why she thought this: did he look at other women? Had he said her age was an issue? No. She said that her aunt had been married to a man who'd left her for his secretary, 10 years her junior, and she'd grown up listening to her aunt and her mother talk about what scoundrels men were. She'd also had dates previously where her age and inability to have children (she'd had a hysterectomy for medical reasons) had been an issue. She was convinced that she'd be left alone, old, and heartbroken as soon as he'd had enough of her.

I convinced her to bring him to the next session. He came happily and described how wonderful it was for him that he'd found such a connection with her. He said that he had never wanted children, and could imagine growing old and sharing their mutual passion for traveling.

When I asked him if he found her attractive, his eyes almost bulged out of his head. He said an expletive, and proceeded to describe in exquisite detail (much to her embarrassment) the parts of her body that were his favorites. I helped her explain her fears to him, and the history that had created them. I then taught them both how to deal with these "gremlins" of hers when they showed up, as well as how to set boundaries with her more cynical friends.

The moral of the story is that even though people often end up with similar-aged partners and some men choose younger women, not all men do. Love – real love – might not be worried about such trivial things as wrinkles. So it might be worth taking a look at your own internal ageism and see how it could be limiting you.

> ### DOING SINGLE WELL: WHAT IS IMPORTANT TO YOU?
>
> Here is a list of qualities you could choose in a future partner. If you could choose any of these qualities in the man you settle down with, which would you choose first? Number them in order of priority, from 1 (for most important) to 5.

- Personal growth and curiosity

- Imagination and creativity

- Humor and fun

- Inspiring others and influencing people

- High intellect

- Spontaneity and flexibility and / or a sense of adventure

- Kindness and care

- Groundedness and stability

- Openness, frankness and / or the ability to communicate well

- Passion and emotional expression

- Honor, integrity, and trustworthiness
- Attractiveness
- Wealth
- Sexual compatibility
- Cultural and / or religious similarity
- Similar dreams and goals
- Similar hobbies and interests

Now, where did attractiveness come for you in your order of priorities? Even if attractiveness rated in your top five, what is the chance that if you took a survey, every single man you surveyed would pick attractiveness (or youth) first? Post your thoughts – or even your experiences of dealing with this issue – on Facebook @doingsinglewell

MYTH 4: THERE'S NO ONE LIKE HIM

Of course, we are all unique, so technically, this thought is not really a myth. However, just because we won't meet anyone exactly like our favorite ex, it doesn't mean we won't ever feel the same way about a new partner.

Now, I'm sure your ex, or the date that you were so hopeful about, had many fine qualities and there were lot of good things happening between you. But think about it: If he didn't choose you, there must have been at least one major thing wrong with him!

I like to think this myth is a by-product of our attachment system, and our evolutionary history. Compared to other mammals, humans are born "premature" – unable to walk or fend for themselves – and are therefore very vulnerable. So, to ensure the survival of our genes, humans have an innate attachment system which results in emotions such as love, and impulses such as proximity seeking – an urge to stay close to our attachment figures.

Indeed, psychologists have shown that babies show preference for their own mothers over a stranger from a very early age, and a mother can distinguish her own baby's cries from others very early on. It is this attachment wiring that also causes separation anxiety and grief when we lose someone we are attached to.

When we pair-bond as adults, our partners become our attachment figures in our attachment brain. Therefore, just like we only have one mummy, and she feels irreplaceable to us, when we break up from a partner, it is only natural for us to feel like no substitute will do.

The really great news is that although it seems like we could never feel the same about someone else, the truth is, we have the capacity to love many people. Just ask anyone who has had their heart broken and gone on to love again!

This myth relies on an unhelpful thinking pattern known as "emotional reasoning" – which means you mistake feelings as facts. The truth is that divorce and remarriage is so common these days we all know someone who has loved and lost and then gone on to love again. And just like those people have, you can be sure that you will always attach and re-attach if you give yourself the opportunity.

A client example for you. Let's call her Ms L (for Loyal):

Ms L came to me after the break-up of her one and only relationship … five years after it! She had met her ex-husband in high school, they had traveled together, built their house together and had their little girl together. They were the couple that everyone thought would be together for ever. That was until he left her.

It had happened very suddenly – one week they were working out who would do pre-school drop-offs and pick-ups, and planning their next family holiday to Fiji, and the next he told her that he didn't love her anymore. She couldn't believe him at first. He'd never complained, they never fought … sure, they didn't have any relatives around to help with childcare, so hadn't had much time as a couple over the past few years, but she'd thought this was normal, and they'd have more time in the years to come.

She'd pleaded with him to go to counseling and he'd refused. He'd moved out the same week, and she'd only seen him to drop off, or pick up their child since then. Every time she asked to talk he'd go quiet on her, or get angry, and tell her she needed to move on. Six months later she heard from a mutual friend that he was living with another woman.

Ms L was sobbing by the time she'd finished this story. She told me about how she'd given him what he wanted in the settlement without argument, and always took his childcare weekends when he wanted to go away with his new partner. She said that she felt she owed it to him. When I asked her why, she told me about how she'd always thought he was too good for her.

She'd been a dumpy bookworm at high school and had been flattered when he'd taken an interest in her. She'd grown to know him as the kindest, smartest, most wonderful of men. Her own relationship with her alcoholic and verbally abusive father had been fraught, and she said that her husband had been the first and only man to love her. Deep down, she'd known he would find someone better and more worthy than her in time.

When I asked her if she'd dated since the divorce, she bowed her head and shook it, 'No.' She said she'd loved her ex with her whole heart and still loved him. She didn't think she could ever feel that way about anyone again. As you can imagine, we spent many sessions working on her self-esteem, and helping her understand how her history of abuse had caused her to feel unworthy of a man's love. Amazingly, and probably through some rather non-therapeutic badgering, I finally got her to download a dating app. Her homework was to like 10 men a day, and talk to anyone who she matched with.

There are rare times in life when a therapist's prayers are answered. In my time treating single women, two lovely ladies have fallen in love with, and married, the first men they matched with. They were both so happy with the beautiful, gentle, and loving men that they'd met on that first date. Ms L was one of them.

DOING SINGLE WELL: MAN MYTHS ON THE RADIO!

The "no one like him" myth is almost hardwired into human's attachment brains. You don't have to look far to see evidence for it in our art and culture. Some of our most popular songs and stories are based on this idea of the irreplaceable soulmate. Turn on the radio or pick up a classic romantic novel and see if you can find the evidence for yourself. (Hint: Adele seems to have hit the "no one like him" myth hard if you listen to a few of her most popular songs!) Post your thoughts on Facebook @doingsinglewell

IN SUMMARY

It is easy when we are feeling discouraged to jump on the man-myth bandwagon and blame the male population for our current state of singleness. However, not only are these myths largely untrue, they are also unhelpful. Blaming something outside ourselves and outside of our control will just leave us feeling more disempowered, demotivated, and desperately dateless.

These beliefs arise as a defense mechanism in single women. They unhelpfully protect us from experiences of vulnerability, rejection, anxiety and loneliness, because they get in the way of being open to men and pursuing a relationship. Doing Single Well means treating all people – those with a penis and those without – as unique individuals, and judging them on a case-by-case basis.

DOING SINGLE WELL: MAN-MYTH BUSTER

Become really aware of your thoughts around men and dating over the next week or two. Notice when any of these man myths come up and try to look deeper. What were you feeling just before that idea popped into your head? Can you identify the discomfort or vulnerable experience that might have produced them? I'll share some more info on how to manage uncomfortable feelings in Chapter 8, but for now, just become conscious of, and compassionate towards, your patterns and process. Post your thoughts @doingsinglewell

Psychologists have found that the following, all-too-common, unhelpful thinking patterns lead to poor adjustment, anxiety, and depression. They will all prevent you from Doing Single Well. Next to each, is an example of how those patterns can be seen in the man myths we've discussed and in the "gremlins" we'll talk about in the next chapter.

Unhelpful thinking pattern	Description	Example
Black and white thinking	Seeing only one extreme or the other	e.g. 'All the good ones are taken.'
Mental filter	Dismissing anything that doesn't "fit" our view of the world, disqualifying the positive and selecting the negative to focus on	e.g. 'All the good ones are taken,' 'All men want younger women.'
Should statements	Thinking in terms of "shoulds" and "musts" can put unreasonable pressure on yourself or others	e.g. 'I should not be so picky,' 'He should want to have sex.'
Personalizing	Blaming yourself for anything that goes wrong	e.g. 'He dumped me because I wasn't funny enough.'
Labeling / name-calling	Making global statements and name-calling	e.g. 'All men are players,' 'I'm unlovable.'
Overgeneralizing	Taking one instance in the past or present and imposing it on all current or future situations	e.g. 'Thinking *all* men are anything!' and 'I'll never meet anyone.'
Catastrophizing	Blowing things out of proportion	e.g. 'I'm over the hill and am going to end up alone with cats.'
Fortune telling	Believing we know what is going to happen in the future	e.g. 'My time is running out,' 'I'll be left on the shelf.'

Mind reading	Assuming we know what others are thinking	e.g. 'He's only interested in one thing,' 'I'm too old for him.'
Emotional reasoning	Mistaking feelings for facts	e.g. 'I feel unattractive therefore he must find me unattractive.'
Magnification and minimization	Magnifying the positive aspects of others and minimizing your own	e.g. 'There's no one like him,' 'I'm not good enough.'

CHAPTER 5

THE SINGLE GIRL'S GREMLINS

What are the gremlins?

The gremlins are the habitual thoughts that sit in the back of our minds. Along with the man myths, these gremlins will prevent us from Doing Single Well. Like the little creatures they are named after, they are mischievous scamps that will pick the exact right time to wreak havoc ...

Just after you get rejected by a guy you were keen on, the "I did something wrong" gremlin will jump out. Just when you hear of a friend's pregnancy, watch out for the "biological clock" gremlin. And just as you are plucking up the courage to talk to a handsome stranger at a bar, you can be sure of an attack of the "not good enough" gremlin.

The gremlins that plague single women can breed prolifically. All we need to do is pay them a drop of attention and then *POW* they're stuck in our head all the time! In the following pages you will read about the common gremlins that plague single women and what to do if you manage to catch one of them inside your head.

Below I've referred to all gremlins as "he" but you can give your gremlins any gender or name you like. Sometimes when the "stuff" that bothers us comes from the females in our life (e.g. mother, sister or friend) it may be more natural for you to think of your gremlins as girls.

The "I'm Too Picky" Gremlin

This little guy is a contagious gremlin. In my experience, he almost always begins by being spread from the mouth of a well-meaning friend or family member. You know how it goes: you go on a date, or two, or three, you might have even been in a relationship for months or years … but no matter how long you've given it, you've decided you just aren't feeling it anymore, and so, you end it. Then, in search of solace and solidarity you seek out the support of friends and family. But, instead of support you get … a gremlin! 'You are too picky,' someone will say! 'You want too much,' 'You'll be left on the shelf!' And as soon as the words are out of their mouth, this nasty little gremlin lodges himself in your head and makes you question your choice.

So how do we know when it's acceptable to take someone "warts and all" as the old saying goes? We all know that you can't go into a relationship expecting to change the other person, so where is that line between "settling" (choosing a relationship out of fear of not having another better option) and being "too picky"? Psychologist Dan Wile said that all relationships are a bag of problems, and the key to a successful relationship is picking the bag of problems that you can live with for the rest of your life. Psychologists John and Julie Gottman spoke about the "four horsemen" that are predictive of relationship failure: criticism, contempt, defensiveness, and stonewalling.

So what this means is that there is a lot of love in saying "No." It is a very kind thing to do to end a relationship with someone who you can't wholeheartedly love and accept as they are. If you find yourself being overly critical or contemptuous of your partner, you are doing them a favor by not allowing them to waste any more time being with someone who doesn't think they are altogether amazing.

'I was desperately trying to like a guy. He seemed like such a nice guy! He was good looking and smart, and he seemed really keen on me, which is always nice! It's just that every time we went out, I couldn't help but be judgey about his clothes … On our second date we met for breakfast at a café near where he lived and he greeted me with a bear hug shortly followed by a proud admission: 'These are my pajamas!' His sandy-eyed, sleep-matted hair and tracksuit that morning set the tone for future dates, and when I started catching myself being catty and sarcastic about his choice in footwear or beer-branded T-shirt, I knew, no matter how superficial that made me, I had to end it.' – Julia, 35 years old.

'She dumped him because of his dress sense?!' I hear you ask. Once again, different things have different value to different people …

Maybe his clothes are a difference that you think you can live with? Great! In this case, try speaking about it with affection: 'Make sure you wear a beer T-shirt! I won't recognize you otherwise!' The Gottman's talk about this as "dialoguing" around "perpetual problems." Perpetual problems are perpetual because often they're about differences between you as people and differences in what your lifestyle needs are. Sixty-nine percent of relationship conflict is around perpetual problems so it's a good idea to try dialoguing!

Or maybe, he truly doesn't mind changing his clothes. That's great too, provided he's not just doing it to make you happy. You don't want to become the nag who is constantly criticizing him. Nor do you want him to make compromises now, that he will resent you for later. If you talk over the things that are irritating you with your date, and find that either of you need to step over your boundaries and do things you aren't really willing to do in order to achieve a compromise (see Chapter 17) then it doesn't matter *what* the deal breaker is, it's a deal breaker.

Some signs you are not being "too picky" and need to end the relationship are:

- Being highly critical of your partner / date

- Finding yourself bored and tuning out from them as they talk

- Rolling your eyes at your partner or sighing at them

- Begrudging the time you spend with them

- Always arriving late and / or cancelling on them if you find something else to do

- Finding your eyes wandering or starting to flirt with someone else

- Complaining about your partner / date to friends

- Feeling annoyed when your partner texts or calls

- Finding your partner doing any of the above when it comes to you!

- Realizing that you have very different dreams for the future

- Having serious problems in the relationship, e.g. conflict that one of you isn't willing to get help for, or willing to work on

- Feeling unimportant to your partner and finding that they aren't meeting your needs despite repeated attempts by you to communicate them

- Feeling scared of your partner or anxious about upsetting him for fear of how he'll respond

- Any kind of physically threatening behavior, feeling pressured to have sex when you don't want to, and any kind of name-calling or yelling

DOING SINGLE WELL: THE BOUNDARY BAGEL (ADAPTED FROM GOTTMAN, 2015)

In order to work out if you are, or are not being "too picky" when dating, you need to understand what are your core needs and in what areas you can be flexible. It is very important that you don't compromise on anything that feels absolutely essential to you and cross your own boundaries.

However, it is also important to recognize that no one will be absolutely perfect for you, and there will always be areas in any relationship where you will need to accept your date's individuality.

Step 1: Consider something that you don't like about your date.

E.g. Julia would say, 'I don't like his dress sense.'

Step 2: Think of the inside circle containing the ideas, needs, and values you absolutely cannot compromise on, and the outside oval containing the ideas, needs, and values that you feel more flexible towards in this area. Make two lists.

E.g. Julia might say:

Inflexible: My date having self-respect, my date having ambition, my date caring for me enough to want to look good for me, attraction to my date, being proud to bring him to social functions.

Flexible: Cost of clothes, style of clothes (neat and clean is enough), whether he chooses them himself.

Step 3: Think about why your inflexible needs or values are so important to you. You may even like to discuss them with your date if an issue like this has come up.

E.g. Julia might say:

'To me your clothes say something about how much you value yourself and your level of ambition. I was always told that you should "dress for the job you want not the job you have." I need to feel you love me enough to want to look smart for me. I value aesthetic, I take special care to make everything look good in my apartment, etc. I also need to feel proud of my partner and confident to take him to social functions with me without fear of others judging him negatively.'

THE "BIOLOGICAL CLOCK" GREMLIN

The "biological clock" gremlin generally creeps up on us in our thirties and grows exponentially over the next decade or so. Similar to the "too picky" gremlin, the "biological clock" gremlin is fed by friends, family, and the stuff we read in the media. If that isn't enough, a visit to your doctor to ask about fertility will be sure to give you a few more facts and figures to make your "biological clock" gremlin grow even stronger!

Of course, the "biological clock" gremlin preys particularly on women who have always dreamed about becoming a mother. This gremlin will be the voice in their head telling them that their "time is running out" and they'll never find someone in time to have a family. He'll be sure to point out all the babies around her, and give her a little jab of pain and desperation every time a friend announces a new pregnancy.

Although women throughout the ages have had to manage the grief of infertility, fertility problems are on the rise, given the trend to delay marriage and family life. It is true that a woman's fertility declines in her thirties to forties. However, it is supremely unhelpful to hear constant internal reminders that "your time is running out." Time, as we experience it, is linear and constant. The seconds will keep ticking by at their usual rate, no matter whether we're battling our gremlins, or out having fun. But being stressed by the "biological clock" gremlin *will* negatively affect the fun we have while dating, as well as our self-confidence, and our hope for the future. It may even lead us to make a poor decision and "settle" in order to secure a family life.

If you have always wanted to be a mother and have reached your mid-thirties, I encourage you to try to compartmentalize "finding a partner" from "having a family." If you desperately want a baby, begin that journey as best you can, providing your finances and life situation allow it, even if you haven't found Mr. Right. Consider if you have steady work, support from family and friends, adequate accommodation, good health cover, and parental leave options . If it seems feasible to do so, it's okay to start a family by yourself – there are plenty of family-oriented people who will totally understand why you made that choice. What is more, any truly family-oriented guy you date after you have your baby won't be put off by it, he might even see your ready-made family as a bonus!

Some tips to arm yourself against the "biological clock" gremlin:

1. Date authentically.

Declare that you are looking for a serious relationship in order to start a family early on in your dating. Say nice "no's" to men who say they "aren't sure" what they want, or they "just want to see how things go" without declaring that they are looking to settle down. You want to be dating someone with clear family goals themselves. So it's totally okay for you to let the men who are ambivalent, or haven't yet gotten to that stage, move on and find someone more suitable. And remember, wanting a family is only one of the things you are looking for in a man! See Chapter 12 for more ideas.

2. Get a fertility assessment and advice from a reputable source.

There is plenty of "data" out there, and it can be hard to separate the fact from the scaremongering. Although it is important to keep in mind that fertility clinics make their business out of the "biological clock" gremlin, you do need to know the facts. It is far better to know than to assume. With knowledge comes choice. If your fertility is uncertain, get to a doctor and get it checked out. Every year, advances are being made in the fields of egg-freezing and related fertility technology, and they are slowly becoming more affordable too. So, you owe it to yourself to at least consider all the options available to you. See it as a biological insurance policy which will somewhat relieve the pressure put on you by the "biological clock" gremlin.

3. Live up the single life.

Too many single women who are family–oriented will give up their weekends to go to their friend's children's birthday parties. They'll give up their nightlife to stay in with their married-with-young-children friends. Although these are very nice things to do on occasion, if you live your life like someone who is married with a family, you will experience all the downside of being a parent with none of the good stuff that makes it worthwhile. Try unfollowing the friends who always post baby photos on their social media if it makes you feel sad. Try saying no to the kids' birthday parties, and encourage your mother-friends to get a babysitter so they can have a night off with you – you'll be doing both them and yourself a favor!

DOING SINGLE WELL: YOUR SINGLE DAYS ARE NUMBERED!

Let's imagine that this will be your last month as a single woman forever. After this month, you will meet the man of your dreams and have all the joys and the responsibilities of a full-time partner. What would you do this month? How would you savor it? Make a list of all the things you'd like to do, and the things you'll miss once you are in a relationship. Then, make yourself a priority and do them!

Feel stuck? Just ask a married friend what she misses about single life – you'll be sure to get a bunch of ideas!

Inspire others and post your list or photos of your single fun! Instagram #Doingsinglewell Facebook @doingsinglewell

---

4. Choose your own adventure.

Remember that if you want it enough, you will be able to have it, one way or another.

We all have ingrained ideas of the order things should happen, which are fed by the heteronormative scripts in our society. However, if you want a family enough and are willing to consider options outside of the traditional, you will be able to achieve your dreams. Not many women start out dreaming of being a single mother, adopting a child, having a surrogate or donor, etc. However, if you ask anyone who has ever gone down these routes, you will be hard pressed to find someone who regrets having the child they always wanted, no matter how it happened.

The "I Did Something Wrong" Gremlin

This gremlin is a master at twisting facts. First date disaster? He'll be there. Even if it was as obvious as it was off-putting that your date's idea of a good time was to regale you with his extensive collection of dad jokes, this gremlin will pop up and say *you* were at fault for the date going badly.

End of a relationship? No matter how it happened, and despite us all knowing that relationships are two-way streets, this gremlin will lead you to believe that there was something you did that broke it, or something you failed to do, that could have prevented the break-up.

It's funny how many lovely ladies will tell me that they weren't that keen on their date, or found serious flaws in their partner, and were ambivalent about continuing the relationship, *until* he rejected them! Rejection seems to be the magic potion that awakens this gremlin. Once awake, this glass-half-full gremlin could focus on how this rejection is fantastic – amazing even – because now you don't have to go through the awkwardness of dumping your date. But instead, he'll just get us to stew on what we could have done differently to save the relationship or get that next date.

So, instead of allowing the "I did something wrong" gremlin to make us feel shame and self-consciousness, throw a party when he arrives! Give him a high-five and celebrate the art of making mistakes, especially if it leads to our dates rejecting us! How else can we tell if a guy can love us unconditionally, and has the skills to go through good times and bad? If a guy is going to cut us off cold at the first mishap or misunderstanding, it's good to know early. How on earth are we going to get to "until death do us part" unless he can talk about what has upset him, or isn't suiting him, so we can work through the issues? Why would we want things to drag on any longer with someone who can't participate in relationship problem solving?

DOING SINGLE WELL: MR. WRONG!

Write a list of all the things you feel you may have done wrong in your last dating experience or relationship. Now flip this list ... if your preferences were the ones we were taking into account, what did your date do wrong? For example, if you wrote on your list "talked to much" then, naturally, he wasn't assertive enough or didn't participate enough in the conversation. If you wrote "spilled wine down my shirt" then perhaps he was humorless and didn't put you at ease, or treat things in a light-hearted enough way to make that feel okay.

Post your stories about your Mr. Wrong on Facebook @doingsinglewell

THE "BAG LADY / ALONE WITH CATS" GREMLIN

This gremlin is a master of "catastrophizing" – making mountains out of molehills (and you can find out more about that in Chapter 4). Ironically enough, one of its favorite stories is how we'll end up alone with cats. A close second favorite is that we'll end up a bag lady, with no one to care for us in our old age. Bridget Jones had a particularly creative gremlin who gave her a fear of "dying alone and being found three weeks later, half-eaten by an Alsatian."

Many single women who live quite happily in the present, fear for their futures. This gremlin particularly likes to target childless single women past their forties. His near cousin targets single women with kids, making them fear for their children's future if they were to die prematurely. The siren songs of this gremlin have choruses like: "old and sick," "lonely," "isolated," "unsupported," "forgotten," "unwanted," and "insignificant." This gremlin is not the life of the party as you can see!

Many single women who have an attack of this gremlin know that they are being irrational – they are often self-sufficient financially, with enough to provide for themselves into their old age. They may even have many friends they could ask for help if they wanted to. However, the beauty of stereotypes is that they don't need to be based on any current reality to have power over us!

In fact, research in gerontology suggests that single women tend to fare very well in their old age – being cared for by their social networks. They say that childlessness has little bearing on happiness, life satisfaction, or loneliness in the elderly, and that having friends is much more important. They also suggest that single women are masters at making and sustaining friendships when compared with other social groups.

So don't let the "bag lady" / "alone with cats" gremlin rain on your single parade! Make a plan for your old age if you have any concerns or uncertainties. But otherwise, don't listen to his whispers, and keep on going about your fabulous life, as usual.

And P.S. Cats are great! As a new cat owner, I think everyone should have one!

THE "I'M NOT GOOD ENOUGH" GREMLIN

I've left the best for last. This is the gremlin of all gremlins. It can come in many exotic breeds. If the "I did something wrong" gremlin is all about errors we make on the date or in the relationship, the "I'm not good enough" gremlin tells us that we *are* the error. You can be sure that, if you have any insecurity, there will be a "not good enough" gremlin lurking at the heart of it. These gremlins love to hide out in the cracks in our self-esteem, no matter what they represent. We could feel not interesting enough and he'll appear. Not successful enough? – even better! Not traveled? Not educated? Not cool? He'll set up home in our heads and put his feet up, feeding on all our self-doubts!

He's a clever little creature. He's got this way of using the "mental filtering" bias (see Chapter 4) to make us pay attention to all the evidence that says our insecurity is correct, and make us ignore all the contrary information that would put holes in his story. (For example, you *must* be stupid if you got that many trivia questions wrong ... who cares that you aced your last exams!)

By far the most common breed of "not good enough" gremlin, is the one that will tell us that we are not attractive enough. It might be that the gremlins say we are too fat, too old, too short / tall, too ugly, our skin is too bad, or there is some specific physical flaw that renders us entirely unappealing. Because we all can find *something* about our bodies to hate on, none of us are immune to him.

What is more, we do live in a very image-focused culture. Image-altering technology and plastic surgery help create a false ideal for women to aspire to. What we see in the mirror just can't compare to what a good filter, a little airbrush, a Botox needle, or a surgeon's scalpel can do! Internet dating technology, with its emphasis on photos, can also be a trap and make single women think that we will only succeed if we look hot. Our sense of attractiveness, and our view of what is and isn't attractive, is such a common roadblock to Doing Single Well that I will address it in Chapter 7.

The "not good enough" gremlin likes to trick us into thinking that attractiveness is something we have or haven't got. What is more, when he has gotten into our heads and told us that we aren't attractive, he then plays a fun game to see how much of our time he can waste by getting us to pursue attractiveness. Whether it's going to the gym, making up our face, buying fashionable clothes, or getting beauty treatments, when these behaviors are done to increase our sense of attractiveness to others they are considered "safety behaviors."

A safety behavior is what we do to compensate for an anxiety-provoking thought ... in this case "I'm not attractive enough." Safety behaviors have the particular effect of easing the anxiety temporarily (e.g. I feel attractive enough going out tonight because I've spent an hour making myself up). But in the long term, they reinforce the anxiety-provoking belief "I'm not attractive enough" because we never get to experience whether people find us attractive just as we are.

Because these safety behaviors work in the short term, we become more and more hooked on engaging in them to give us relief from feeling unattractive. This is how people end up spending large amounts of money on beauty treatments and getting increasingly extreme things done to themselves surgically. However, in the long term, they prevent us from getting feedback that people like us just the way we are. Sure, it's nice to have 40+ people like a highly filtered and airbrushed photo of you on Instagram, but having your partner tell you that you are beautiful when you are just waking up in the morning is an experience that few would trade for all the Insta-praise in the world!

Another way of responding to the "not attractive enough" gremlin is to give up and not put any effort into our looks or appearance. Although it may sound like the women who do this are enlightened souls, that isn't necessarily the case. If it's done in the spirit of "it doesn't matter, nothing I do will make a difference" it will be just as unhelpful as painstaking primping. This is because these women no longer see the gremlin for what he is (just a thought in our head) and believe what he is saying entirely. The gremlin has won!

DOING SINGLE WELL: ANTIDOTES FOR THE "NOT ATTRACTIVE ENOUGH" GREMLIN

Many people have had an experience where their view of attractiveness (about themselves or someone else) has been proven to be subjective and changeable. The "not attractive enough" gremlin just likes to try to make us forget these experiences, so we believe he is telling us the truth. To reconnect with the experiences you have had about how beauty is in the eye of the beholder, have a think about the following questions:

1. Have you ever experienced someone getting more attractive to you as you get to know them better? (Or less attractive if they are not nice people?)

2. Have a think about your girlfriends' partners – would you have chosen those guys for yourself? What does this say about varying taste in attractiveness?

3. Have you ever looked back on old photos and become aware of how good you looked in hindsight, while still remembering that you felt ugly or fat when the photo was taken?

4. Collect photos of some of the people you would consider the most attractive celebrities in the world, then survey a group of your friends and ask them who they think is the most attractive out of them. What are the chances that they will all pick the same person? What does this say about attractiveness?

Post your thoughts and observations to help others on Facebook @doingsinglewell or pick a celebrity you find attractive and do an Insta-poll on who agrees #doingsinglewell

CHAPTER 6

BEFRIENDING YOUR "NOT GOOD ENOUGH" GREMLINS

Just like any strongly held belief, no amount of positive affirmations or mantras tend to make a dint on a "not good enough" gremlin infestation. It's like trying to clean your house with a handy-wipe! So what do we do about them?

... We get to know them, and develop an affection for them!

What?!

Yep, you got it. If you can't beat them, you can at least try to see the humor in them!

Although it seems a little crazy, befriending your "not good enough" gremlins will reduce their influence in your life. You will find that you start to feel as nonplussed about them as you do when there are clouds in the sky. You don't welcome them, they may even be inconvenient. But they aren't a disaster, or even anything that deserves too much of your attention. Below I will guide you through a step-by-step process to befriend your "not good enough" gremlins so that they loosen their grip over you.

1. WHAT DO YOUR GREMLINS TELL YOU?

The first and most important step is to make the invisible, visible. Every minute we have dozens of thoughts, and it is in this constant thought-stream that the "not good enough" gremlins dump their poisonous messages. So, the first task is to work out what your gremlins are saying to you specifically. Here is one way to do that:

Perfect Girlfriend Material

A) Who is perfect girlfriend material in your eyes? If a guy could date anyone, what sort of woman would he choose? Think about someone you know who you think would be the "ideal girlfriend /

date" in a guy's opinion, and write out why you've picked her. Or, just write out a list of qualities that you think a guy's ideal girlfriend / date would have.

B) Write out a list of your own actual qualities, or better yet, get a close friend to write the list. If you were to be scrupulously honest on an internet dating profile, how would it read?

C) What are the key differences between your list of idealized girlfriend / date qualities and your description of who you actually are? Odds are, your gremlins will lurk in those gaps.

'My best friend was the super-star of our school. She was pretty and popular. She was the head of the hockey team, valedictorian of our school, and the belle of our high-school formal. She had long blonde hair, long legs, and a perfect smile. All the guys wanted to be with her. I'd even have some guys trying to be friendly with me, just so they could get closer to her. I was like the comic-strip sidekick; the only attention I got was because I was friends with her. It was awful being in her shadow. At times I wanted to end the friendship, and even asked my mum once if I could change schools! But I couldn't hate her, she was just too nice! I remember going to bed in high school praying to God that he make me funny and kind and pretty and smart, just like her.' – Lucy, 29 years old.

2. WHERE DO YOUR GREMLINS COME FROM?

Now that you have an idea of what your gremlins tell you specifically, it's time to work out how they got into your head in the first place. To do this, think back to the earliest memories you have of feeling that you are not enough in your specific way.

Alternatively, think about how your gremlins make you feel, then focus in on that feeling for a minute or more ... How old does that feeling seem to you? Can you remember the first time you felt like that? Write the history of your gremlins, just like these ladies have done:

'I'd never been self-conscious as a child. I had a pretty average body and there wasn't a lot of bullying at my school. It was only when I got to high school and everyone around me started to hit puberty that things changed. Where other girls were developing boobs, I remained as flat as a pancake. I wouldn't have minded so much if it wasn't for the guy I had

a crush on. We were friends and I longed for him to notice me as more than a friend. I remember one night, we were hanging out at a party, and someone joked about us "lovebirds" sitting together. I still to this day remember the face he pulled as he said to them, 'Haha, Kate's so flat she could be one of the boys! As if anything would happen there!' – Kate, 40 years old.

'I was never very good at school. In first grade our teacher had a system where we had to sit in order of smartness. I was put at the end of the dumb row. She would constantly ask me to answer questions in front of the class and I would go blank, feel hot, and never have any clue what to say. The kids would laugh, and I'd wish for a hole to open up and swallow me. I wasn't diagnosed with dyslexia until high school.' – Mel, 37 years old.

'I was always a chubby kid. Our whole family was on the larger side and it bothered my parents a lot. I remember going on a soup diet with my mum when I was 7 years old. I remember going to Weight Watchers and weighing in with all the older ladies, at 10 years old. I never had confidence to talk to boys in high school because I was sure I was too fat for them to take notice of. I thought that if I tried they would tease me. I remember having a crush on a guy and being terrified that anyone would find out. I felt so unworthy of having those types of feelings as a fat girl. It's funny now because I remember a couple of guys asked me out. At the time, I thought they were making fun of me, but now I wonder if it was genuine and I was just too damaged to believe it.' – Fiona, 27 years old.

3. APPRECIATING YOUR GREMLINS

Hopefully you have been able to trace your gremlins back to some experiences which help you understand where they came from. So now, let's find out why they developed and what purpose they served.

Because humans are social creatures that live in "packs" or communities, it is important for us to be liked and accepted by others. Because we don't have sharp teeth or big claws to defend ourselves in the wild, early humans found safety in numbers. Being kicked out of the tribe meant certain death in the time of dinosaurs! As such, our brains developed all the wiring we need for attachment and interpersonal skills. This "mammalian brain" is responsible for our social responses and also the fear we have of criticism and rejection from our social group.

In order to prevent criticism and rejection we developed what Freud used to call the superego, what is commonly referred to as the inner critic ... and what we are now calling the "not good enough" gremlins. This internalized voice criticizes you in an effort to prepare you for any external criticism you may receive – if you already know your haircut is awful, it doesn't hurt so much when someone laughs at it. As discussed in the last chapter, the gremlins will have you either surrender to your fate (e.g. 'I know I'm ugly so I'm not going to even put myself out there to be rejected') or engage you in safety behaviors to try to change, or cover up your perceived inadequacies (e.g. 'I'll let him do all the talking, that way he won't realize how boring I am').

So, believe it or not, your gremlins are actually very well intentioned. One might even say they are trying to look after you, and stop you from being rejected! The only problem is that most of our gremlins are outdated. They were useful when they first sprang to life, to deal with the difficult experiences you were going through at the time. But for most of us, this danger has now passed, and the people who criticized us as kids are largely gone from our lives. In cases where we do still have some critical people in our life, being an adult means we will often have better ways to deal with these people than letting the "not good enough" gremlins put us down before they get a chance!

Well-meaning as your "not good enough" gremlin is then, we need to gently move him aside, so we can deal with things in more empowering ways.

'I know where my low self-esteem comes from. That voice in my head even uses the same words that my sister used to. When I look in the mirror, it is as if she's talking to me from inside my head. 'Four eyes and freckles, what boy would want you?!' Joking about it made it easier somehow, it had become something of a running joke in our family. When someone asked me why I was single, I'd joke that my sister got all the good genes and my fairy godmother got lost in transit. Now I know how unhelpful buying into all that was. And every day I roll my eyes and stick my tongue

out at the sister-in-my-head, and blow a kiss at myself in the mirror... freckles and all!' – Vanessa, 28 years old.

What can you do to relate to your gremlins differently? How can you befriend them, while not believing what they say to you? Next time they come up, try one of these things until you find one that works for you:

- Thank your gremlin for that thought and remind yourself that it's just your gremlin, not the truth.

- Stick your tongue out, roll your eyes, blow a raspberry, or flip your rude finger at your gremlin when he pipes up.

- Affectionately remind your gremlin that his job is done, and he doesn't need to keep popping up for you now. You are a grown-up and you've got this.

- Remind yourself that your gremlin is an internalized version of someone who hurt you in the past and affectionately tell that person to get out of your head, e.g. 'Bugger off, Dad, get out of my head and go play your golf!'

- Try singing what your gremlin tells you to the tune of 'Happy Birthday' or changing his voice so he sounds like Mickey Mouse or Donald Duck.

- Try mixing up the words of what the gremlin says as many different ways as you can. 'Enough I'm Good Not,' 'Good I'm Not Enough,' 'Not Enough I'm Good.'

- Try listing out all the experiences you have had that belie what the gremlin is telling you ... or ask a friend to help you for a more objective list!

- Take a moment to feel compassion, and comfort the part of you that was small and vulnerable when the gremlins were born. Give yourself a hug, or stroke your own arms gently as if you were comforting a small, frightened animal ... tell that "inner child" part of you not to worry about the bad gremlins. They aren't real.

No matter what you do, don't criticize yourself, or get frustrated with yourself for having your gremlins; that just makes them worse. Your gremlins are there because that was the only way you could cope with what you experienced at a younger age, and criticizing yourself for being self-critical will just compound the problem!

4. WATCHING OUT FOR GREMLIN BOOBY-TRAPS

Because your gremlins want to protect you from rejection they will booby-trap you in one of two ways:

1) They will have you avoid putting yourself in the position to get rejected, or

2) They will have you overcompensate, and do things in order to mask feeling "not good enough"... If you can cover up your flaws, no one will reject you!

As we spoke about before, neither of these behaviors are a good solution for building confidence and Doing Single Well. This is because when you do these things you never get to embrace experiences where you are liked for all your perfect imperfection!

AVOIDANCE

Think about it ... do you avoid things, or put anything off because of your gremlins ...

- Do you avoid dating, or put it off until you reach some standard of "good enough" (e.g. avoiding dating until you lose weight)?

- Do you avoid telling a crush that you are interested in him?

- Do you avoid being honest about what you are looking for in terms of a relationship?

- Do you avoid telling a date you'd be interested in seeing him again?

- Do you silence yourself, or hide some parts of yourself? Do you keep your story, your needs, or your feelings hidden? If you think you might be an avoider, there is more for you in Chapter 9.

'I would never tell a guy I was dating that I have two cats. I don't want to be seen as the "crazy cat lady"! I've even avoided bringing guys home, just so they don't have to find out!' – Ella, 38 years old.

'I've put off dating for the last 10 years. Every New Year I make a commitment: This year, I will go on a diet and lose weight and then I will

feel comfortable dating. It's not that I haven't had guys interested in me, but I can't believe they would be interested in anything long term with me looking like this.' – Cassy, 45 years old.

OVERCOMPENSATION

Also think about the efforts you go to in order to fit in, or be attractive. The "not good enough" gremlin is especially fond of picking women whose self-esteem is dependent on other people's approval. This means that if you have a case of the "not good enough" gremlins, you may find yourself focusing on working out what kind of girl your guy wants and pretending to be that person. Laughing at his bad jokes, eating his spicy food, even *groan* going to the cricket! What have you done to prove that you are his ideal girlfriend?

Similarly, you can look for any efforts you make to be "perfect." How much do you edit the texts that you send him? How long do you spend getting ready for dates? How often have you gotten sexual before you were really ready to, just to keep him interested?

Now, of course there will be times that you do things for yourself. For example, you might begin a program at a gym in order to lose weight so you can feel better in your body. You might want to get a stylist to create a wardrobe for you, or get a nice haircut. You might want to enroll in a course, or take up a hobby. If it is done for *you* (not for *him*) then go right ahead ... just make sure you don't put off dating while you are doing any of these things. Remember, you are good enough for him without the frills. ☺

5. AIM FOR CONNECTION AND AUTHENTICITY, NOT PERFECTION AND ATTRACTIVENESS

Instead of trying to be the perfect date and working hard to make yourself as attractive as possible, laugh when the gremlins tell you that you aren't good enough. Remind yourself you are just perfect for the person who is perfect for you. The next chapter will be all about how connection creates attraction, and authenticity is magnetic, so you are actually working towards your gremlin's end-goal of not being rejected. You've just found a better, more proactive strategy of your own!

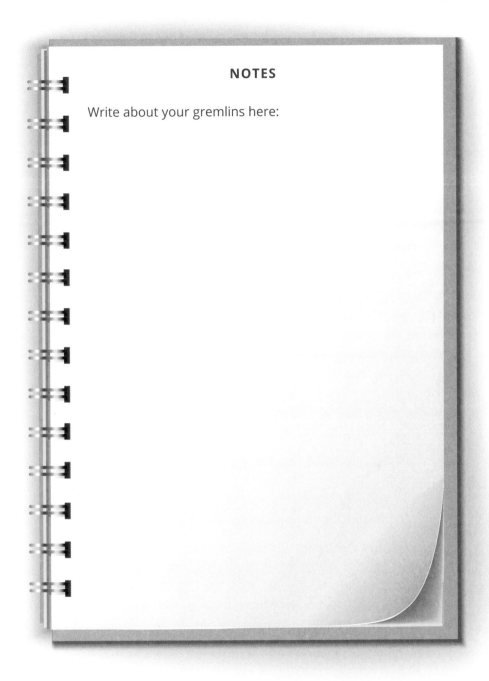

NOTES

Write about your gremlins here:

CHAPTER 7

WHAT IS ATTRACTIVE ANYWAY?

We all want to be attractive. We are all likely to be flattered if a guy finds us attractive. We have all yearned to be more like our attractive friend that everyone seems drawn to.

We may not like it, but there is a reason why our society has such a thriving beauty industry – psychological research shows that physical attractiveness is important. Physical attractiveness influences many different aspects of human social interaction. For example, people preferentially date, mate with, associate with, employ, and even vote for physically attractive people. People also tend to automatically ascribe positive personality characteristics to physically attractive individuals. This is often referred to as the attractiveness halo effect, or the beauty-is-good stereotype.

Researchers speculate that the appeal of attractiveness has got to do with survival of the fittest, and how we are wired to be drawn to people who have characteristics that indicate superior genes and fertility, and healthy immune systems.

However, if you've never considered yourself classically attractive, there is no need to worry. What people view as attractive isn't just highly subjective; it is changeable. Attractiveness, in a purely physical sense, actually counts for very little in dating when all factors are considered equally. Read the research findings below with a sense of humor and watch out ... Whether you are familiar with these points, or you have absorbed other messages about what is attractive or not, we all tend to think that what we view as attractive is what everyone views as attractive. We unhelpfully elevate our subjective opinions to the position of objective truth!

Here's what "the research" shows makes a woman physically attractive:

THE TOP FIVE OF FEMALE ATTRACTIVENESS:

1. **Attractive faces:** Nice faces are more important than nice bodies for men who want long-term relationships and conversely, hot bodies are more attractive for men who are looking for something short term! So what makes a face attractive? Symmetry and feminine characteristics such as big eyes and "well-proportioned" lips (approximately 50% the width of your face!).

2. **Waist-to-hip ratio:** Although men do prefer bigger breasts, having close to the ideal waist-to-hip ratio (where your waist is around 70% the circumference of your hips) counts for more in terms of attractiveness.

3. **Hair and teeth:** Healthy hair and white, evenly spaced teeth are found to be more attractive ... There is mixed evidence as to whether hair length matters.

4. **Being like his mother:** Men are more attracted to women with the same hair and eye color, and the same height as their mothers. Also, men who are born to mothers over 30 years old are more likely to find older women more attractive.

5. **Height and arms:** Taller women are rated as more attractive if they have legs proportionate to their height and long arms!

I know, right?! I'm sure by now you're starting to realize why it is ludicrous to place so much stock in our appearance. Who'd have thought arm length would make a difference?! And how are you going to know if you look like a guy's mum?

Putting some eyeliner and some lippy on, and investing in some good conditioner can't hurt (particularly if it is done to please yourself as part of your own self-care ritual). But none of us can control the symmetry of our face, or how tall and long armed we are! The great news is that research has shown that behavioral qualities make much more of a difference in attractiveness than physical features.

THE TOP SEVEN SEXY BEHAVIORS:

1. **Wearing red**

2. **Ovulation!** Apparently men are subconsciously aware of pheromones and other natural ovulation cues.

3. **Voice pitch:** A moderately high pitched and slightly breathy voice is perceived as more attractive. Conveniently, women who are talking to a man they find attractive will unconsciously speak in a higher pitched voice.

4. **Head tilt:** When a woman tilts her head forward enough that she is looking slightly up at a man, it is perceived as more attractive.

5. **Grooming:** Neat and clean grooming and good posture are shown to be just as important for attractiveness as fixed features like height. Moreover, men prefer women who are more "natural" looking and wear up to 40% less makeup than the average.

6. **Being outdoorsy:** Men are attracted to women who took what the researchers called "hunter gatherer" risks – activities and dangers similar to what our ancient ancestors would have faced. Modern day examples include skiing, mountain climbing, white water rafting, and other outdoor activities. Taking modern risks, like drug taking, and not wearing a seatbelt are not considered attractive.

7. **Laughing at his jokes:** It's hardly surprising that men like women who laugh at their jokes. The proviso I'm going to put on this one is only if the jokes are funny! You don't want to end up with someone whose potty humor you find repugnant … so it could be really beneficial if you aren't attractive to those guys!

Interesting, yes? But not the stuff of compelling research!

So, it's fine if you want to go out and buy yourself a red dress, and a nice cleanser. But beyond that, I don't suggest you pay much attention to the other items on the list. Going out on dates only when you are ovulating is not going to make for a great social life, and if you go trying to change your voice, and exaggerating your head tilt, you'll likely come out sounding like Minnie Mouse and give yourself a neck cramp!

I also don't suggest you make yourself outdoorsy if your idea of a good time is a couch and a book. Remember, intimacy is all about getting to know someone's inner world. If you pretend to like outdoor adventures, then you might just end up with an outdoorsman who doesn't know the first thing about you … And think of all the dreaded camping you'll have to do!

'I put on my internet dating profile that I liked the outdoors – it seemed to be what everyone else was writing on theirs. A great guy asked me on a hiking date ... It took hours and I ended up sunburned, sweaty, bug eaten, and cranky. The guy never asked me out again, and I was relieved! Ever since then I've been much more real on my profile, and the dates I have been on have been surprisingly fun.' – Laura, 29 years old.

So, if it's not about how we look, or what we do, then how do we become our most magnetic selves?!

I'm so glad you were wondering! Like baking a good cake, attractiveness comes down to the quality of ingredients. Good quality, nourishing ingredients lead to a tasty, satisfying, and moreish cake ... or date! In this model, the ingredients are what you put into the date on a personal level – how you show up; how you pay attention; how you relate, and the personal qualities that you demonstrate.

GEM'S SURPRISINGLY SIMPLE ROMANCE RECIPE

1. Authenticity

Authenticity is the ability to know and stay true to ourselves, even in the face of disapproval. Authentic people are open and unguarded, and are able to communicate their emotions honestly and freely.

Brené Brown, my therapist-crush and the researcher who put authenticity in the spotlight, describes authenticity as "a practice of letting go of who we think we're supposed to be and embracing who we are. The choice to show up and be real. The choice to be honest. The choice to let our true selves be seen." If you want to read more about authenticity, I highly recommend her book *The Gifts of Imperfection* (2010), and have a peek at Chapter 17!

Intuitively, we all know that warm, down-to-earth, honest people are magnetic. Research also supports that men who are looking for long-term relationships prefer someone who seems honest ... it even affects their judgment of physical attractiveness; honest women are perceived as more fit, healthy, and kind.

2. Attunement

Attunement is a kinesthetic sensing – meaning a non-verbal way of responding to another's rhythm, emotional state, and experience.

It is our felt sense of how someone is, rather than what we know or learn about them through what they say. Like ballroom dancing with an expert partner, good attunement is felt by both people as a sense of unbroken connectedness, resonance, and a feeling of being in sync.

Our ability to attune comes down to how present and responsive we can be moment-to-moment to another person's emotional needs and moods. For most people this happens largely unconsciously when they are focused in an undistracted way on another person.

Not everyone is a natural at attunement, but it is something that we can practice until it feels natural, just like if we keep practicing the steps of a dance, we'll eventually forget the steps and just dance. So, for people who don't find attunement so easy, there are a couple of shortcuts:

1. Relaxing and focusing attention: When you calm your body down, your racing mind will generally follow. When you are on a date, make the effort to slow your breathing down and relax any tense muscles. Start with your shoulders. Like a golfer about to tee off, small physical adjustments like this can help us enter into what sports psychologists call the "flow" state – a state of full immersion, involvement, and enjoyment in the process of an activity.

2. Leaning in and mirroring: We have a natural urge to get closer to people we find attractive. Leaning in to your date shows that you are interested in him, and conveniently, research shows that men are attracted to women who are interested in them. Mirroring involves loosely copying your date's body language – touching your hair shortly after he does, smiling when he does, etc. Research has found when you mirror someone they perceive you as more attractive and likeable.

DOING SINGLE WELL: GET AN A+ IN ATTUNEMENT

Go to a café and watch people interacting with each other, or look at people on TV. Can you pick the people that have good attunement with each other? They will look like they have known each other forever, like their bodies are almost in sync. Attunement happens even in our earliest relationships, so you might like to notice how different mothers are attuned to their babies. Notice how individuals in a group of people attune to each other. Can you tell who is attuned to who in the group? You might even be able to see the patterns shift over time?

Post your observations on Facebook @doingsinglewell

3. Connection

Ever wondered why sometimes, you just click with someone? But other times, the date just feels off – you don't warm to the guy, and you don't feel like you have much connection?

John and Julie Gottman are renowned couples researchers who have extensively studied what makes a successful relationship. Although they mainly study established relationships, knowing what makes for a good relationship can be very useful for singles!

In every interaction there is a possibility of building connection and trust, or turning away. In fact, the Gottman studies show that happy couples make as many as 100 bids for connection over the course of a single meal! A bid is any gesture – verbal or non-verbal – for some sort of positive connection. A bid can be a request for conversation, humor, affection, support, or simply attention.

Conceptualize every time we relate to someone as a bid for attention: every text, every Facebook post, every call or email, every glance or smile, every question or statement. How the other person responds to that bid for attention will determine how secure, comfortable, and validated we feel, and thus how much we click with that person. There are three ways to respond to a bid:

1. Turning towards:

HIM: 'Oh look! Taylor Swift is coming on tour!'

YOU: 'That's great, hon, she's your favorite, right? We should get tickets.'

2. Turning away:

HIM: 'Oh look! Taylor Swift is coming on tour!'

YOU: (Distractedly) 'Huh? ...' (Continues to look at iPhone and doesn't engage.)

3. Turning against:

HIM: 'Oh look! Taylor Swift is coming on tour!'

YOU: 'You are such a dirty perv! Only teenage girls like Taylor Swift, not grown men!'

As part of his research, Dr. Gottman conducted a study with newlyweds and then followed up with them six years later. The couples that stayed married were much better at one thing: turning towards bids for attention. In fact, couples that stayed married turned towards one another 86% of the time. Couples that had divorced averaged only 33% of the time.

Based on this, if you look at happy couples or, in our case, good dates, we will turn towards our date (and he to us) in a 5:1 ratio. We don't have to worry about being perfect, but we do have to be wary of advice to play it cool. And we have to be careful of indulging any bad habits we have developed in using "negging" (teasing criticism or put-downs) to ease our anxiety in a dating situation.

"Turning towards" actions metaphorically deposit goodwill into the relationship's emotional bank account. Research shows that the act of turning towards leads to even more turning towards. It's a positive feedback cycle. And, there is no need to be disingenuous and overly gushy; responding with kind awareness is just as effective as an enthusiastic proclamation: *'I'd love to talk about your mother!'*

Turning towards is the more verbal component of the non-verbal attunement we described above. In other models, it has been called "responsiveness" (e.g. Reis, Clark & Holmes, 2004). A responsive partner makes their date feel understood, validated, and cared for. Responsive partners pay attention when their dates share their perspectives (rather than "turning away") and ask questions to gather more information, or to better comprehend. They will make their date feel that their perspective is valid, even if they hold a different perspective (rather than "turning against"). This makes their dates feel respected and supported.

DOING SINGLE WELL: CONNECTION QUEEN

If you think that you might need practice in attuning and connection, enlist a close friend or family member. Tell them you are working on the way you connect with people and ask if they are willing to help you out. If they agree, don't tell them exactly what you will be doing, but let them know that after your interaction, you'll ask them to give you a rating out of 10 on how connected and comfortable they felt with you. And tell them you want them to be honest!

During the interaction, relax yourself and practice mirroring their non-verbal behaviors. After a short lag, do something similar with your hands to what they have done, shift your body or legs in a similar way to them. Lean in and out in flow with them. Try not to be too obvious or robotic, aim for gentle and rhythmic, like a dance.

You can also practice turning towards bids. Respond with interest to the things your friend is saying; try not to get distracted, interrupt, or criticize them. Try to make your friend feel understood, validated, and cared for.

To see if what you are doing is having a real effect, try your attuning and mirroring every second time you interact with this person. You should find a big difference between the scores you get when practicing the new interactional style from when you are just being "normal," if you are changing the right things.

Post your experiments on Facebook @doingsinglewell

TRUST YOUR GUT

We often get a sense of poor attunement without really realizing why we are feeling uneasy, or not interested in our date. Trust yourself! Don't blame yourself for being "oversensitive" if you start to feel anxious when he doesn't respond to your texts.

Don't tell yourself you are being picky if you barely got a word in on a date – our feelings are our hardwired responses, and a great source of information about how things are going, and how well our date is able to relate to us! We *all* deserve to feel happy and good in our relationships, and there is no point settling for someone who can't make you feel connected.

Do remember though: Treat him as you'd like to be treated. To give him the best chance of correcting any bad habits he has developed, or bad dating rules he is following, it's always good to tell him what you need from him first, rather than just dumping him cold. Giving the warning, 'I need you to respond to my texts if you still want to see me' or saying, 'I seem to know a lot about you now, I'm wondering if you are interested in hearing about me?' – isn't that hard, is it?

4. Positive personality traits

Studies have shown that almost all positive personality traits impact on how attractive a man views a potential partner. Qualities like kindness, respectfulness, openness, agreeableness, assertiveness, and a positive attitude are all more important for attractiveness than body type.

In one study (Swami et al., 2010) there was no significant difference in the body type a group of men rated as most attractive when they rated pictures alone. However, when they received positive personality information, in addition to the pictures, they rated a far wider range of body types as more attractive. Conversely, when men were given negative personality information, they rated a far narrower range of body types as attractive, showing that non-physical cues have a big effect on perceived physical beauty.

The same is true for facial attractiveness. One study (Zang, Kong, Zhong & Kou, 2014) had participants look at pictures of faces and rate them for attractiveness and found there was no significant difference in attractiveness ratings. Two weeks later, they rated the faces again, but this time they were given positive, negative, or no personality information relating to the faces. Results showed that the faces with the positive information were rated as significantly more attractive than the faces with no information, which were rated significantly more attractive than faces with negative information. These were the same faces as before!

Finally, the cross-cultural study we looked at in Chapter 1 (Buss, 1989; Buss et al., 1990) asked 10,047 people across 37 cultures, which of 32 possible characteristics they desired in a long-term mate. Many characteristics were universally desired by both sexes. Worldwide, women and men wanted mates who were intelligent, kind, understanding, dependable, and healthy.

DOING SINGLE WELL: THE TRICKS OF THE TRAITS

In the table below, there is a list of the positive personality traits that the research shows are attractive to men.

Looking back on past dates or interactions with friends, think about how you might determine whether your date or friend had these positive qualities. What did they do that made you think that?

Make a list of the behaviors you identify and use this as a guide for your own dating efforts to come!

Post your behavior lists to help others @doingsinglewell

Positive Trait	Description	Examples – put your own here
Kindness	Being caring, thoughtful, generous, understanding, and considerate	e.g. Asks me how I'm feeling
Respectfulness	Being courteous, tolerant, responsible, reliable, dependable	e.g. Turns up on time
Authenticity	Being self-aware, genuine, open, honest, assertive	e.g. Shares his history freely

Agreeableness	Being warm, tactful, optimistic, cooperative, encouraging	e.g. Makes an effort to cooperate to find plans that suit us both
Insert your own here:		

5. Eye contact and smiling (the icing on our attractiveness cake!)

Brain imaging techniques allowed researchers to find that viewing attractive faces causes more activity in the brain's reward centers than viewing unattractive faces does. However, all faces were found to be more rewarding when they were smiling, and when they were looking at the viewer. Because someone looking at us, or smiling at us, indicates that they are probably interested in talking to us, these findings suggest attraction is not only influenced by physical beauty, but is also influenced by how interested a person appears to be in you.

Smiling naturally makes us more attractive to a guy. The even better news is that smiling at our date, even if we have to fake it at first, can improve both our moods! Studies have shown that people who fake a smile – particularly a "Duchenne" smile that involves their eyes as well as their mouth – report improved mood, and have signs of reduced stress. What is more, thanks to "mirror neurons" in our brains, emotions are contagious: your smile will likely lift his spirits too, so you'll both have a better time!

Hopefully you can see that physical attractiveness is far less important than what our image-obsessed culture makes it out to be. What is important is how you interact, and what your interactions say about you and your interest in your date.

CHAPTER 8

CRAZY, LONELY CAT LADIES

There is no doubt about it, being single can come with its fair share of yucky feelings. So can being in a relationship, but let's face it, when you are in a relationship at least you can blame him for your miserable feelings! Many single women complain of experiencing unpleasant feelings as a result of being single, irrespective of whether they identify as generally happy or unhappily single. Often though, the difference between those who are Doing Single Well and those who aren't is simply how they manage these feelings.

Loneliness is the biggest culprit that sneaks up on single women when they are supposed to be enjoying their me-time. The temporary state of loneliness provides fertile ground for a gremlin attack and shame spiral which can drop us all the way down into a black hole of depression. Once depressed, we are then steeped in the feelings of disconnection, sadness, hopelessness, and worthlessness that come with it. We may be sitting at home on a Friday night feeling a little lonely or bored and then *WHAM!* All of a sudden, we have a head full of gremlins telling us that we're losers who will be alone forever!

Anxious worrying is also endemic among single women. It can show up with depression, or by itself. Worry is future-based negative thinking – the "catastrophization" we saw in Chapter 4. Worry often occurs when there is uncertainty and general pessimism. Not having a committed relationship gives wonderful freedom to single women, but the dark side of that equation is that life is often more uncertain. Combine that uncertainty with everyone-and-their-dog saying we'll die lonely cat ladies, is it any wonder that worry shows up?!

'I keep having dreams about being old and sick and alone ... shuffling around my apartment in the dark, and sitting on my couch staring out the window at all the people out there going home to their families ... couples walking hand-in-hand. I just worry I'm never going to meet

anyone ... and I'll become one of those sad old people that die alone in their apartments only to be found months later due to complaints about the smell.' – Miriam, 31 years old.

THE LOWDOWN ON EMOTIONS

Before we start talking about specific feelings that occur for single ladies, it's useful to have an understanding of feelings generally. Although it sounds obvious, feelings are sensations in your body that occur in response to a trigger. Sometimes the trigger is external to us (e.g. watching a tear-jerker like *The Notebook*) but often the triggers are our thoughts. Although it is possible that some emotions precede thoughts, most of the feelings we'll be discussing in this chapter will be amplified, if not triggered directly by our thoughts, particularly those pesky gremlin thoughts we discussed before.

Thoughts are *not* feelings although the two are often experienced together. This is an important distinction, because how we work with our unhelpful thoughts is different to how we manage the feelings they produce.

Feelings are also *not* permanent. A lot of the distress that single women experience with their unpleasant feelings is because they catastrophize: because they are feeling bad now, they worry that they are going to feel like this forever, or at least until they are in a relationship!

Doing Single Well involves recognizing that having a range of feelings, both good and bad, is a natural part of life. Even being in a relationship won't guarantee only good feelings! We've all had the experience of going to bed feeling low and waking up in a better mood. It is important that no matter what we are feeling at any one time, we remember that this feeling – however inconvenient – is temporary. Like rain clouds in the sky, it's a bit of a bummer, but not a disaster! And, just as we wouldn't let a spot of rain ruin our day, it's important not to let any negative feelings that come up for us interfere with our plans and dreams.

Many people try to avoid or get rid of painful feelings. This is not necessary, and in some cases is actually unhelpful. Common examples of avoidance include:

- Numbing (Netflix marathon anyone?)

- Opting-out of situations where unpleasant feelings arise – like avoiding going on a date

- Drinking alcohol

- Going on shopping sprees

- Bingeing on your favorite foods

In the next chapter, we'll deal with avoidance in more detail.

 The best thing to do when unpleasant feelings arrive is to care for ourselves as we work through them. This is different from trying to fix them or run from them. You don't expect a warm bath and a cup of tea to cure a cold when you have one! But when you're sick, you still care for yourself in this way because it comforts you. Thinking about how we would care for a sick child can give us some good ideas of the types of things that are likely to help comfort ourselves during difficult emotional experiences. Usually these things are tactile or sensual things that feel good, for example:

- Take a warm bath with scented oils.

- Dim bright lights, light some candles, burn some scented oils, and put on some enjoyable music – treat yourself as if you were a treasured guest.

- Put on your most comforting pajamas or trackpants, and wrap yourself up in a cozy blanket.

- Give yourself a massage with nice moisturizer, or give yourself a manicure, pedicure, or facial.

- Cook yourself some comforting hot soup, or a favorite meal, set the table nicely and eat by candlelight.

- Buy or pick yourself some beautiful flowers, put them where you'll see them often and allow yourself to admire them.

- Sit in the warm sunshine and read a good book or magazine.

- Go for a gentle walk and sit in a park watching the world go by, or lie on your back in the grass, and make shapes out of the clouds.

- Try a gentle yoga or Tai Chi class – watch it on YouTube, and you won't even have to leave your living room!

- Get your favorite takeout for dinner and eat it while watching a funny movie.

- Make a list of your special achievements, no matter how small they may seem.

- Buy a coloring book and some pencils and do some coloring in. Or, buy some wool and teach yourself to knit or crochet via YouTube.

If you have a little more time and energy, you could:

- Go for a drive somewhere scenic and stop for a picnic.

- Get a professional massage, facial, manicure, pedicure, or a new haircut.

- Visit a museum or art gallery, and give yourself the time to browse at your leisure.

- See a good movie or live show, alone if need be.

- Wake up early and watch the sun rise from a good vantage point, or find a favorite spot to watch the sun set.

- Go through your wardrobe. Give away any clothes that don't flatter you, and arrange the remaining clothes neatly.

- Buy yourself a treat of new clothes, shoes, makeup, or perfume, or just enjoy a leisurely window-shop.

- Visit a zoo and enjoy finding out about all the animals.

- Feed your inner child – go to a playground to swing on the swings or find a trampoline to bounce on.

- Take a swim at a beach or a local pool, or have a spa or a sauna.

- Go bushwalking or hiking in nature.

- Play some dance music and dance around by yourself or try a dance class.

- Clean your jewelry and begin to wear it again. Or clean out a long-overdue cupboard and only keep the things that give you joy.

- Go for coffee and cake at your favorite café.

- Buy a plant and choose a lovely pot to plant it in, or a perfect spot in the garden.

- Put some of your favorite photographs into frames and put them on display, or frame a favorite piece of art.

- Play with an animal – and if you don't own a pet, visit a pet-loving friend.

- Pretend to be a tourist in your own town and explore the attractions.

You will have noticed that all of the things above are things we can do by ourselves. It isn't that going out and meeting up with friends is a bad way of managing negative emotions, but it can lead to distraction from those emotions, rather than healthy processing of them. Making ourselves frantically busy and scheduling our weekend diary so that we don't have a single minute to feel anything is not Doing Single Well. (Using the guideline above, you wouldn't make a sick child do that!) We all have to learn how to enjoy our own company, and show up for ourselves in a caring way.

DOING SINGLE WELL: NAME IT AND TAME IT (ADAPTED FROM HARRIS, 1999)

This is a technique of getting to know your feelings and managing them better, using mindfulness. You may remember that mindfulness is a way of paying attention in an accepting and non-judgmental way. Bringing mindful attention to your feelings will reduce the impact and influence your unpleasant feelings have on you. When feelings aren't experienced as roadblocks you'll be free to do things that can help towards making a meaningful life, in a way that a Netflix marathon or a bottle of wine can't.

The acronym "NAME" will help you remember the steps:

- Notice

- Acknowledge

- Make Space

- Expand Awareness

1. Notice

When strong feelings show up, the first step is simply to notice them. Take a few seconds to scan your body from head to toe, and zero in on wherever the feeling is strongest. Notice where the feeling starts and stops. Where are its edges? Is it at the surface or deep inside you? Is it moving or still? What temperature is it? Some people are more visual, and it can help to ask yourself: If the feeling was a color or a shape, what color or shape would it be? Would it be smooth, spiky, etc.?

2. Acknowledge

Once you have noticed the feelings and sensations in your body, the next step is to openly acknowledge their presence. Studies have shown that just labeling emotions can help you regulate them. Say to yourself: 'Here is a feeling of anger' or 'Here is a feeling of insecurity.'

3. Make space

We can learn to become more accepting of strong feelings if we give them plenty of space. This is the opposite to the urge to "get rid" of them. Try breathing in deeply and imagining that your breath flows into and around that feeling in your body. And as it does, imagine that a hollow of open space is created inside you. The breath is cushioning your feeling, your body is opening up, or making room for all those unpleasant sensations. See if you can allow those feelings to be there, even though you don't want them. You are simply giving them permission to be present.

4. Expand awareness

The final step is to expand awareness. In other words, reach out and make contact with the world around you. As you do this, your feelings are still present, but you have made room for them. They can hang around until they decide to leave. Meanwhile, you are free to act and do the things that will help you live a good life, whatever that means for you. Don't wait until you feel better. If there is something meaningful or important you could be doing, then do it right now.

Post your attempts and observations on how "Name It and Tame It" works for you @doingsinglewell

THE BIG L

L stands for loneliness – the emotional social pain response to perceived isolation. Loneliness usually includes anxiety about lack of connection with other people, and a sense of hopelessness about future connection. Just like a feeling of hunger, we have feelings of loneliness to help us meet our survival needs. Because humans don't have big claws or teeth, we only survived as a species because we moved about in groups. We developed feelings such as loneliness to ensure that we were motivated to connect to a group when we found ourselves alone. Therefore, just like a rumbling tummy motivates us to seek out food, loneliness motivates us to connect with others.

The interesting thing about loneliness is that it is both genetic and subjective. Although twin studies indicate that the tendency to feel lonely is partially genetic, it is also highly subjective in that there is no one set of circumstances which necessarily produces loneliness, and not all people feel lonely in the same situation.

Loneliness isn't just the bugbear of single women – people in relationships and marriages, and those who have families can all experience it. Loneliness is therefore not the state of being alone – some people experience solitude without loneliness. Loneliness comes more from having a gap between our desired levels (or type) of social interaction and the levels we actually have in reality. Stephanie Dowrick in *Intimacy & Solitude* (2014) suggests that a person enjoys solitude when she is comfortable with herself and secure in her social connections. She holds on to these connections in her head even when no one is there.

The seemingly obvious solution to loneliness would be to pick up the phone and connect with friends. But research has shown that treatments that target negative thinking are more effective for loneliness than those which provide opportunity for social interaction … once again it's all about what's going on in your head!

DOING SINGLE WELL: LETTING GO OF LONELINESS

You'll find that your thoughts when you are lonely fit into those unhelpful thought categories we looked at in Chapter 4.

For example:

'I'll never meet anyone' (fortune telling)

'Everyone else is busy' (overgeneralization)

'Nobody cares' (mindreading)

'I'm a loser' (name-calling)

'My other single friends are way more popular and busy' (mental filtering)

It's important when you are alone that you don't just sit there and stew on this kind of thinking. Being alone does not mean you have to feel lonely. Follow this sequence next time loneliness is knocking on your door:

1. Do you want to have company or to go out? If 'yes,' have you contacted everyone and asked if they are free to do something? If no one is free today, make a plan for when they are next free.

2. What can you focus on if you stay in? Do you have a book, a movie, a podcast, a game, or a hobby you can give your attention to? Remember, we don't want you to be sitting on the couch with an empty mind because that is when the unhelpful thoughts will buzz in!

3. Remind yourself that this is just a temporary feeling that will pass. Do the NAME strategy.

4. What can you do to be kind to yourself tonight while you feel this way? Pick something off the self-care list above and nurture yourself through it.

Post how you let go of your loneliness on Facebook or post a photo of yourself enjoying your solo time #Doingsinglewell @doingsinglewell

CRAZY CAT LADY

The "crazy cat lady" archetype was around long before the Simpsons, or the DC Comics villainess, Catwoman. Whereas dogs are referred to as man's best friend, cats are associated with women, particularly single women. It's thought this is because, when first domesticated, dogs were given specific tasks like hunting or guarding which required them to be outside with the men. But cats were ratters or mousers, and kept inside the home where the women worked. A cat lady may also be an animal hoarder. Interestingly, recent research has linked a cat parasite *Toxoplasma gondii* with psychiatric conditions, including hoarding, the inference being that these so-called crazy cat ladies were actually victims of a parasitic infection!

Pet therapy has long been a treatment for loneliness and depression. Interacting with pets for only 5–20 minutes has been shown to have a greater and faster effect on lowering stress levels than medication. There are a great many benefits of having an emotional bond with a pet if you don't have a large social support network. Older people living alone are four times less likely to be diagnosed with depression if they have a pet.

Embracing being a crazy cat (dog / hamster / rabbit / guinea pig) lady may be a good way to help you become a satisfied single woman!

SHAME

- Shame is that feeling you get when someone asks you, 'Why are you single?'

- Shame is what causes you to avoid online or formalized dating channels, or deny you are dating online for fear of being seen as "a loser."

- Shame is that feeling that spreads through you when he doesn't call … And even though you weren't that into him, you're still upset.

- Shame causes you to tell your friends (if untruthfully) that you are not interested in a relationship so that they don't pity you for being single.

- Shame is the favorite emotion used to taunt you by the "not good enough" gremlins.

SHAME IS THE FEELING THAT YOU ARE UNLOVABLE

Shame to me is that wash of hot or cold over your body; the feeling of your heart in your throat; your breath stopping; your stomach sinking; the "cringe moment"; the feeling that makes you want to hide your head in your hands, or just disappear.

Shame is experienced slightly differently by everyone, but is a universal emotion designed to protect us from social rejection. Remember, social rejection was a real danger for early mankind because, as pack animals, we had so few abilities to survive in the wild by ourselves!

We respond to feelings of shame in one of three ways:

Moving away: We feel like hiding, withdrawing, and keeping the shameful thoughts or experience a secret. Shame is one of the most debilitating emotions because we often don't talk about shame. As such, we feel unique and alone in our unlovability, like we really, truly are flawed and hopeless.

Moving towards: We try to "make good" through people-pleasing and appeasing ... To fit in, to "be cool," to change ourselves into a more "lovable" version. Not only is this hard work and inauthentic, it is unsustainable. Ultimately, it traps us in a cycle of thinking that says the only way we can be lovable is to be perfect, and then compels us to work hard to make others like us.

Moving against: We try to gain power over others by being aggressive or shaming them, in order to fight our own shame. This is what motivates bitchiness and meanness.

'I remember ending things with a guy I'd been on three dates with. He seemed like a nice guy but I wasn't feeling it, so I told him that I'd had fun, but I felt we were too different. I was stunned when he got super angry with me and said that he didn't have fun, and that he was only dating me to try to help me with my emotional problems and "serious issues"!'
– Kristy, 37 years old.

When we don't know how to helpfully manage shame it can be disastrous to Doing Single Well! At best, we put on a good front to try to make people like us, or to try to get the guy, but that only makes us feel anxious and fraudulent in the process ... It's all too easy to think: if they only knew the "real me" they wouldn't give me the time of day. At worst, we become hamstrung by our shame, and remove ourselves from dating and / or living a good single life.

SO, WHAT DO WE DO ABOUT SHAME?

Well, the good news is everyone is unlovable ... A little bit. Ask any long-term happy couple and they'll tell you with affection about all their partner's flaws.

Love, in the real, felt sense, is not the pursuit of the ideal. Love is just a helping hand, a series of biological reactions in our brain that generates the feelings and motivation to help us overcome the difficulties. When you find someone who is open and ready to fall in love, he won't mind that you are carrying a few extra kilos, that you have a quirky sense of humor; or that you haven't yet achieved everything you wanted to. He will love you in your glorious imperfection and hopefully be patient while you struggle to do the same!

A *helpful* response to shame:

1. **Identify** when you are in shame. Learn how your body responds in shame so you can recognize it when it happens.

2. **Take time out**. Do not talk, text, or type during the height of shame if possible. We can often give a knee-jerk response that we will regret later (moving against) or that will perpetuate our low self-esteem (moving towards).

3. **Soothe**. Lower your physiological arousal. You can do this through slow breathing or gentle self-touch (e.g. cuddling, rocking, stroking yourself like you would comfort a baby). Slow breathing lowers your yucky-feeling adrenalin and cortisol levels, and gentle touch stimulates the feel-good chemicals of endorphins and oxytocin.

4. **Common humanity**. Remind yourself that everyone makes mistakes, is imperfect, and feels shame (even the guy you are dating, and that happily married friend you might wish you were)!

5. **Be kind**. Replace the self-critical thoughts from the "not good

enough" gremlins with kind thoughts – the sorts of things you would say to a friend, or a small child if they came to you feeling bad. Being real and believable is important to make the kindness stick. No mantras please! Instead, acknowledge any mistakes – but without the name-calling and sneering at yourself. For example: 'It feels really bad that he doesn't want to date me anymore, but it doesn't mean I am worthless, just that we are looking for different things. Most people experience this at some time in their life.'

6. **Share**. Shame loves secrecy (hence the moving away response). As soon as possible "confess" your shameful scenario or gremlin thoughts to someone you know will give you the validation and empathy that you need. Remember to select your audience carefully: The only thing shame loves more than secrecy is judgment!

DEPRESSION

When loneliness, gremlins, and shame combine and are left to fester too long, the result is often depression. Depression is an unrelenting low mood which involves frequent feelings of sadness and tearfulness. Some people experience agitation, irritability, and poor concentration when depressed. Most people report a relative lack of energy, lack of pleasure in life, feelings of hopelessness, worthlessness, and guilt. People who are depressed will often report feeling like a failure, and that life is not worth living. When people are depressed they will often withdraw from social activities, and will find that the things that they used to enjoy doing are no longer fun. Changes in appetite and sleep patterns can also signal depression.

Depression can be a serious illness, so if you feel you could be depressed, I urge you to see your doctor or find a psychologist to speak to who will help you through this tough time. Depression is very curable, but the nature of depression is such that, in order to beat it, we have to do the things that are the very opposite of what we feel like doing. However, in life, in dating, and especially in depression, decisions should be made based more on the outcome we want, rather than how we feel.

As a starting point, I encourage you to make sure you are going out with friends at least once or twice weekly, even if you don't feel like it, or you worry that you will be a bore. Research also suggests it is important to increase your exercise at this time, so aim to do some form of exercise for 30 minutes, 3–4 times a week.

Because depression involves hopelessness and inertia, a great many depressed single women I've met have given up on dating. The problem is that although we know we may not meet someone if we put ourselves out there, there is a 100% certainty that we won't meet someone if we stay at home on the couch. It makes sense that, if you don't feel you are lovable or worthwhile (thanks to the "not good enough" gremlins) you will also think that no one could find you attractive or interesting. But just remember: *You* don't have to find yourself attractive or interesting! *He* does! So rather than worry about what you think is wrong with you, you'll be far better off focusing your attention on getting to know more about him. You'll have a better time, and you'll be better company if you do.

If you are dating, well done! *Do* practice the attractiveness recipe in the previous chapter. But *don't* trick yourself into thinking that spouting your man myths and letting your gremlins out to party is showing him the authentic you. Telling a guy all about your perception of "men!" *insert contemptuous tone* doesn't show much consideration to the poor guy giving you his time. Nor is it very useful to make him listen to stories about your ex. (That's your "there's no one like him" man myth at work!) Or to tell him how hopeless and boring you are. (There's your "not good enough" gremlin coming out to play.) Or to apologize for every little thing you do. (That'll be your "I did something wrong" gremlin.) No matter how loud they are, or how frequently they pop up for you, your gremlins are *not you!* So if you find that they try to stowaway on your dates, practice being aware of them, smiling at them (or giving them an imaginary middle finger), but let them go and refocus your attention on attunement and connection. There will be time to reveal all your deep insecurities and vulnerabilities as your dating progresses. We just need to make sure you are doing it with self-awareness (see Chapter 17 for details).

WORRY

Worry can happen to anyone, and at all times of life. It occurs when the future is uncertain, and we find ourselves making up horror movies in our heads. As such, it is a common experience for single women. Although worry is often expressed as a "What if?" e.g. 'What if I'm alone forever?!' most of the time, our emotional state will make it feel as if our worries are truths that *will* occur.

Many people think that worrying will help them plan for, and perhaps even prevent, future negative events. But research shows that worry is not equivalent to problem solving, and people that worry are not any better at dealing with negative events when they arise. They've just experienced the negative emotions twice! The first time when they worried, and then again when something bad actually occurred.

If you are prone to worry, the best thing you can do is become aware of that tendency. When you notice yourself experiencing worry, separate your predictions for the future (the unknown) from what is going on in your life right now (the known). Then ask yourself, 'What can I do right now (if anything) to improve the chances of things going well for me?'

For example:

Sarah was worried that when she went to her cousin's wedding her relatives would ask her why she was still single in front of everyone – and it would feel humiliating. When she thought about what she could actually do about this, she texted her aunt, with whom she was close, and asked her to spread the word to other family members that her relationship status was not up for discussion.

Jane was constantly worried that she would never meet anyone and never have the family she'd always dreamed about. All her friends were getting married and having babies, and it seemed like she was falling more and more behind. So Jane sat down and made a list of all the avenues she could think of to meet new men, and set herself a goal of going on one date a week. She also messaged a friend who'd had her eggs frozen to meet her for coffee so she could get the lowdown.

CHAPTER 9

AM I AVOIDING?

'I'm not sure if I even really want a partner? Isn't it okay to be single? Who needs men anyway?' – Kate, 38 years old.

'I haven't been on a date all year... It would be nice to have someone, but it just seems like too much effort!' – Emma, 27 years old.

'I would love to have a boyfriend, but life is so hectic, I just don't think I have the space to explore something new...' – Meghan, 32 years old.

'I have a great life, a fabulous career, I don't need anything extra ... if only I could get out of the habit of bingeing every night, I'd be totally happy!' – Natalie, 34 years old.

'I've dated heaps of guys, but none of them were "the one." I'm waiting for someone really special and I won't settle!' – Pauline, 40 years old.

Can you tell which of these ladies is avoiding dating and which are genuinely happily single?! I suppose the first question is:

IS IT POSSIBLE TO BE HAPPILY SINGLE?

Remember when we talked about the conflicting "research" in Chapter 1? Well here's some more. You can find studies that say:

• People in long-term relationships are happier than singles

• Only men in long-term relationships are happier than singles

• Single people are happier than people in bad relationships

• Any type of connection makes people happier (not necessarily romantic relationships)

• Marriage doesn't affect happiness beyond the first year or two

Bella DePaulo (2015) poses a number of methodological flaws with research in the area, and suggests we have been misled with all the research and reporting that married people are happier.

Aside from the research there are many theories that would supposedly have you believe that coupling (and related to this, having children) is an important human achievement. The evolutionary theorists suggest that the essential task of humanity is to pass down our genes to the next generation. The old developmental theorists, such as Erikson, saw it as the developmental task of adulthood to find intimacy, or risk isolation. Psychobiologists will cite the many mechanisms and chemicals in our bodies that serve bonding, attachment, and sex purposes as evidence we are supposed to pair-bond. Mirror neurons help us relate to others; oxytocin makes cuddles pleasant; dopamine helps us fall in love. We are wired to connect ... but we are also all born with an appendix – an outdated (if not dangerous) organ – which suggests to me we can't always believe what our biology tells us is important!

Just as we need to understand the social pressure towards heteronormativity, it is important to understand that science and journalism may also fall victim to bias. DePaulo refers to this as "system justification theory" – the premise that there is a psychological motive in the social sciences to defend and justify the status quo so that we can gain a sense of security, legitimacy, and confidence in our lives. So, if we are to leave research and theories aside, we may once again be better taking an individualistic approach. It is up to each individual to determine which path, be it staying single or entering into a relationship, will lead to most happiness and fulfillment for them.

HOW DO I TELL WHAT IS RIGHT FOR ME?

In a culture which pushes us to couple, it is hard to know what is genuinely right for you. If you feel like you would be happy single there will be plenty of times you may question your choice, e.g. when you see a happy couple, speak with a well-meaning but single-averse relative, or come up against one of the difficulties of being single. And if you think you want to get married and have babies, how do you know you haven't just foreclosed and unquestioningly accepted the influence from the people and society around you?

I think the clearest way forward is through looking at your values and dreams.

Our values are the things that we believe are important in the way we live and work. They (should) determine our priorities and will most likely be the measure we use to tell if our lives are turning out the way we want them to. When the things we do match our values, we generally feel content. Values and goals differ in that "to get married" is a goal – and we can check that box – whereas "intimacy" is a value. It doesn't matter how many romantic dinners we go on, we'll never be able to check the intimacy box; it will take life-long work for each of us to continue to meet that value.

Our dreams include "what we want to be when we grow up," but they are bigger than our career. Where do we want to go? What do we want to accomplish? What problem do we want to solve? What hero do we want to meet? Our dreams aren't simply about the things we want to do, but also the person we want to become. Our values are generally embedded within our dreams. For example, no one ever dreamed of climbing Mount Everest without valuing challenge or adventure.

> ## DOING SINGLE WELL: WRITE YOURSELF A LETTER FROM THE FUTURE
>
> One of the easiest ways to connect with your dreams and values is to imagine you are celebrating your 80th birthday. Imagine life has gone rather well and things have turned out just the way you wanted them to. Write yourself a letter telling the story of your life, the opportunities you've had, and the choices you've made. Imagine what needed to happen to leave you feeling so happy and fulfilled on your 80th birthday.

Sample letter:

Wow! What a ride! Who'd have thought so much would have happened to little old me by the time I turned 80! I went from uni straight into an apprenticeship with a large publishing house. Working myself up through the ranks was challenging at times but I loved the learning and really respected my mentors. I couldn't have been more proud making Senior Editor by the time I was 40 years old. I met and fell in love with a wonderful man. We were perfect for each other as he loved hiking too, and so weekends and holidays were spent exploring all the beauty that nature had to offer. We moved in together and got two dogs – our fur babies were the delight of our lives and certainly kept us healthy and active. We bought a little cottage on the edge of the National Park and we've moved there now. The local town is cute, and the people are lovely – everyone looks out for each other. I joined a writers group here and they have become my closest pals – they'll be coming to my birthday bash tonight! Every week we meet over coffee and discuss our latest plot lines and characters – it's a blast!

> To determine what your values are from the dreams expressed in your letter, ask yourself: What is important / meaningful about having achieved this goal or done this activity? In the example above, she might have said things like "growth and learning," "recognition," "connection with nature," "fitness," "companionship."
>
> Post your letters to inspire others on Facebook @doingsinglewell

SIGNS OF SELF-DELUSION

Hopefully we now have a fairly good understanding of our dreams and values. The next trick is to take an honest look at our current actions and choices, and see if they are in line with those values and would logically lead us towards achieving our dreams.

Shame and anxiety can lurk in the subconscious of any lovely lady and are the most common culprits of avoidance. No matter how dressed up and rationalized our reasons are, it's important to examine any areas where our actions and our dreams don't match to see if we are being really honest with ourselves.

For example, if you value intimacy and partnership and dream of getting married and having babies, but are currently single, you should:

- Date regularly (once per week, to once per fortnight at least)

- Not be in any casual, friends-with-benefits, open or one-night-stand type of arrangements

- Not put off dating until you lose weight, work gets quieter, etc.

- Not be in regular contact with your ex (unless you have to, because of the kids)

- Be open to new channels to meet someone if your existing ones aren't producing any good candidates

If your actions don't match your dreams and values, it's time to stop and think about what's stopping you. Avoidance can take many forms and often contains gremlins, so see if you relate to any of the following:

I never meet anyone.

Often 'I never meet anyone' is actually code for 'I'm not willing to put in the effort to go out of my comfort zone to meet anyone.'

I fully agree that internet dating is not for everyone. In fact, in my experience, every single woman must go on her own journey to discover ways of meeting new men that suit her and her lifestyle. Pushing yourself to do something that really doesn't work for you is only going to make you feel unduly negative about the process. Moreover, this negativity will sabotage your chances of being open minded and making a genuine connection.

However, ladies ... the pizza boy is not going to be your Mr. Right!

That's right, staying home and ordering in is a guaranteed way to never meet anyone. So, what are you going to do to further your quest?

Those of you who aren't as keen on internet or speed dating might like to try some of the less dating-focused social sites. Check out some of those sites that aim to bring together groups of people who, like yourself, might want to do some new things and meet some new people. You can attend an activity someone else has organized in your local area, or try organizing one yourself.

Other strategies include asking friends to set you up, or invite you out when they are seeing people you may not know. Organizing a dinner party or an outing where everyone has to bring someone new is also a fun way to go. Beyond that, doing a course can put you into repeated contact with new people, but it can also be a big waste of time if you end up being stuck for weeks with people who weren't your sort from week one!

Dr. Phil of *Oprah* fame also talks about going to a "target rich" area (McGraw, 2007). Think about the sort of guy you want to meet and then make an effort to hang out in places that he would likely hang out. Now, we can deduce that the man of your dreams is probably not going to hang out at your local crochet club, but don't write off making new girlfriends out of your strategy ... Remember, every new girlfriend you make is someone new for you to go out with, and a great source of lots more new people to meet.

It should happen naturally.

Now, I would love for everyone to be the star of their own chick flick and just happen to bump into their partner in the cereal aisle of the supermarket, but that is just not everyone's story! Even single women who have diligently tried all the avenues we've discussed may still not have any luck, despite hours and hours of investment. So, if you have a fairly active social life and are always meeting new people, but not finding Mr. Right, then you'll need to consider other options.

Of course, your experience of meeting men will be culture and circumstance specific: I've heard that, in Italy, men will practically run you down the street to ask you out ... maybe Italian women can wait for it to happen "naturally"?! In the USA, I also hear that men are more bold, and will approach women in a bar, or on the street (something that is practically unheard of in Australia). Whether this is urban myth, one person's experience, or representative of a real cultural difference, I'm not sure. What I am sure of is that if you don't personally have the experience of meeting men "naturally" then being overly invested in the belief "it should happen naturally" is very unhelpful!

If the prospect of more formal dating makes your stomach churn, try examining the source of your resistance. Many single women still carry a sense of shame in being single, and feel that online dating might mark them as a "loser" (that'll be the "not good enough" gremlin at work again!). Some single women have heard horror stories, or had their own bad internet dating experiences that have put them off. Some ladies just hide behind the idea they want it to happen "naturally" because the thought of being proactive and seeking out dates (on the internet or otherwise) fills them with terror. No matter which one of these you are, I don't want to hear excuses, I want to see a full dating schedule! You are not a loser; just because a bad thing happened once doesn't mean it will happen again, and we all know that dealing with anxiety gets better with practice. Don't debate, just date!

No one asks me out!

Some single women will protest that they do keep an active social life and have internet dating profiles. But then they use the fact that no one asks them out to justify their man myths and their gremlin thoughts. All the good ones are taken, right?! I'm just not pretty enough, right?! No! That just does not make sense! I mean, think about it … are you and your friends always attracted to the same guys? Each of us are attractive to, and attracted to, different types. Evolution encourages diversification of the gene pool in this way, so we don't run the risk of dying out as a species. There'll be guys out there who think you're a hottie!

If you are on the internet, start by getting an honest friend to look over your profile. Do you have nice photos? When you message, are you talking about yourself in an authentic and self-affirmatory way? Beyond this, you might need to look at your own likes and selection criteria. Are you being too narrow and assuming too much about the guys you are selecting (or not selecting!) based purely on their photos, or a small bit of profile text? The internet is a great way to meet people if you have the right strategy. Check yours out by comparing it to the guide in Chapter 18.

Sometimes people tell me they're putting themselves out there and going out a lot, but they still don't find anyone approaching them. If that's you, try changing venues, going out with a smaller group of friends (so it's easier for someone to approach you), or, if you see someone you like, approach them yourself. Easier still, try the "Three Second Rule."

DOING SINGLE WELL: THE THREE SECOND RULE

Usually I find that if you are going out, but still not meeting anyone, it has to do with your interactional style – specifically, lack of eye contact!

Men are people too and, yes, they're filled with lots of the same anxieties as single women. Yet, a lot of you will expect that, just because you're out in a bar with your friends, that should be enough of an indication that you are available and want to meet someone ...

NEWS FLASH! You have to show signs that you are open to being met! Sustained or repeated eye contact is the best, least intrusive, and least scary way to do that!

So next time you are out, practice making glances over at the guy you are interested in until they make direct eye contact with you. Then, keep your gaze focused on him for three seconds (with a smile)!

Post your stories about trying the three second rule on Facebook @doingsinglewell

But I'm waiting for my crush to notice me ...

Well, while you're awaiting, time is a ticking! If he really is that special, have you thought of actually asking him out? Go on! Challenge your "no one like him" man myth! Anxiety is a bitch, but the short-term nausea of telling someone you'd like to date them, or the sting of the rejection you're afraid of, is nowhere near as painful in the long term as waiting for someone who doesn't even know you're alive. Remember, even though rejection smarts, opening up to it is the smart choice because:

• You paid him a compliment – who doesn't like being told they are hot!

• You have freed yourself up to meet someone who thinks you are just as amazing as you thought that idiot was!

I'm enjoying a casual thing right now.

Now, I'm the first one to say that women should have as many privileges as men in their sex lives if they want them. The problems occur if:

1. Secretly you are hoping that the casual thing you've got going will turn into something else, or

2. It gives you just enough to make you a little lazy and demotivated when it comes to getting out there and dating more relationship-ready men. Keep in mind that, every night you spend with your friend-with-benefits, you are *not* meeting your Mr. Right.

But I'm still in love with my ex!

This topic is covered in wonderful detail in the book *It's Called a Breakup Because It's Broken* by Greg Behrendt and Amiira Ruotola-Behrendt (2006). In summary, you broke up because something about your relationship was broken. Unless you and your ex are currently actively working through your differences with a counselor, pining for the past is denying that there was something wrong, or denying that you are the only one who really wants to fix it.

Although it can feel like he is the only one for you, staying stuck in that man myth will only lead you to "desperate and dateless" territory. Do yourself a favor and break off contact with him (unless you can't because of the kids). And, if you feel you need to, seek professional counseling so you can process your feelings about the break-up and move forward.

I'm just waiting to be skinnier / to have more time / to make my big break / to do my traveling / to get my promotion / for my kids to grow up ...

There are as many reasons to put off dating as there are single women, and not all reasons are bad ones – so long as you aren't on the relentless self-improvement bandwagon. (Remember you are lovable just as you are – no more listening to those "not good enough" gremlins!) I'll have to leave it for you to judge what your current priorities are. Every second of every day we get to choose where to focus our attention and what to invest in. By all means, you can prioritize your work, your exercise routine, your friends and family, your band, your pet, smoking weed, caring for a loved one, developing an Instagram following ... the sky's the limit! But just make sure that whatever you choose, you do it consciously. Each of those little seconds will add up to your life story, and if you never get around to dating then I want you to make sure you know why, and actively chose it to be that way!

I'm waiting for my soulmate.

Believe it or not, we have feminism to thank for the romantic notion of a soulmate. The feminists of the 1970s began to propose the idea of a relationship based on love, fidelity, emotional intimacy, and best-friendship as an alternative for the power imbalance they saw in heterosexual relationships.

The idea is appealing. Modern life is busy. Modern dating is exhausting. So who doesn't want to believe things should be easy and "predestined." However, I caution you to see this as a type of avoidance. We all know that relationships require work, so it is natural that this can apply even to just getting into a relationship. Also, we all know that no one is "ideal" or a "perfect match" for us ... and if you are in any doubt about that, we'll talk about it more in Chapter 12 ...

Kay Trimberger, in her excellent book *The New Single Woman* (2005), suggests that the idea of waiting for a soulmate gives a defense to single women who desire a relationship but whose situation precludes it. She also suggests women who prefer staying single use the idea of not having found their soulmate to excuse their choice and manage other's opinions.

I suggest that if we want to be in a relationship and our situation precludes it, we should put some problem-solving effort into how we can reorganize our priorities and fit in more dating, rather than get caught up in the fantasy of waiting for our soulmate. Similarly, if we are happy being single, then, rather than fall in line with societal pressure and give lip service to fairy tales, I suggest we may find it far more liberating and fulfilling coming out as single (see Chapter 10).

I have baggage ...

Okay, single women don't usually come out and say this. Instead it will generally sound like:

'I don't want to feel smothered or controlled.'

'I don't trust myself to choose well.'

'Marriage is a passport to misery.'

'He'll just cheat on me or leave me.'

'I don't want to feel tied down.'

Whatever your particular worry, overgeneralization, or fortune-telling fantasy is, these all amount to: '*I have baggage!*'

Life isn't always kind to people and there are baddies out there. Whether we have had our own bad experiences, or we are drawing on the experiences of our friends and family, our brains are designed to learn from these experiences and protect us from future hurt. Anxiety and shame are emotions the brain produces to stop us from getting hurt again. Getting stuck in anxiety, shame, and negative thoughts is pretty effective in preventing more negative relationship experiences ... but it will also stop us from having good ones.

We can't change the past, but we do get to decide what we want to do with it. Rather than giving up and going into hibernation, I strongly urge you to see your history as what it is – over and done with – and with the help of a counselor, if needs be, work on moving past it. See if you can give life and relationships another chance. The information in this book is designed to be a good first step in this process and Chapter 17 talks about how you can own your "stuff" so you can be real in relationships – in all your perfect imperfection. Your past does not have to define you, nor does it have to limit you, so it's time to stop using it as an excuse!

I hate dating! It's too hard! I can't be bothered.

If you think about anything that you have done that was a long-term investment (buying a house, saving for an international trip, getting a degree, etc.) there were bound to have been plenty of steps on that journey that sucked! And in the same way, we are not going to like everything that is involved in finding a partner – makes sense, right?!

We have all been misled by Hollywood movies and romantic novels that sell the idea that if it is meant to be, it will just happen. Dating can be hard, but it can also be a lot of fun. What is the difference between someone who sees it as too hard and someone who sees it as fun? Stop and have a think about how you are perpetuating the "too hard" version …

'I used to think that dating was the pits! I'd spend hours getting ready, agonize over what I'd talk about, and then afterwards, spend the next week dissecting every little thing about the date and coming up with every reason in the book for why he hadn't called. For such a lot of time and energy it just didn't seem worth it. Then when I moved interstate, something changed. I had to get to know my new colleagues and make friends anyway, so I just started to be friendly to people indiscriminately … some of those people were men, and before I knew it, I had guys asking for my phone number and taking me out. After that, it just didn't seem like a big deal anymore!' – Debbie, 30 years old.

Yes, dating takes time and some degree of effort, no matter what attitude we bring to it. But something as important and life-changing as finding your life partner (if that is your dream) has got to be worth a bit of hard work, surely?

So, check yourself for your "there are no good men" myths, ditch the "not good enough" gremlins and get hustling!

DEFINITE SIGNS OF DENIAL

How do you know if you're in denial? Sometimes, single women might suppress or reject the idea that they want a relationship due to the pain or angst that accepting that fact causes. Denial sits deep, and can occur even if you think you know that you don't want to be in a relationship. It is very easy for single women to experience denial about their wanting to be in a relationship if they haven't had success in relationships in the past, if they don't feel worthy of a relationship, or they feel hopeless or anxious at the prospect of dating. Even if you *don't* think this is you, look out for the following signs:

1. **Manic Positivity:** Are you so, so, so happy with your single life? I mean #lovelovelovelovemylife happy? Hmm, perhaps your extreme cheerfulness is trying to mask some not-so-nice but normal aspects of being single … or some normal desires to be in a partnership.

2. **Irritability:** Do you get grumpy and snap at people for no reason (and it's not that time of the month)? This could be related to many stressors in your life, but it's worthwhile stopping to ask if the stress of having unmet needs in your romantic life is leaking out in this way.

3. **Denigration:** Do you tell yourself that you couldn't care less about being in a relationship, and that having a partner is of little value to you? Sometimes this can be an authentic representation of your dreams and values, but sometimes "the lady doth protest too much!" and it is a sign that you are denying your relationship needs.

4. **Bitchy-McBitch-Face:** If you find yourself constantly judging and criticizing your married-with-kids friends, complaining about their choices and bitching about their boring lives, then yep, you are probably secretly envious, and in denial of your own yearning to have some of what they have.

5. **Defensiveness:** Do you become overly defensive when anyone asks about your relationship status? Do you find yourself snapping and eye rolling and getting huffy, even though you know deep down they were just trying to make conversation? Perhaps your defensiveness is an auto-response to a pain-point about being single. Perhaps you do actually want to be in a relationship.

6. **Cynicism / Despair:** Have you just given up and can't be bothered anymore? Does the prospect of ever finding anyone feel utterly hopeless? Do you get sarcastic when you speak about dating? Have you shut off and resigned yourself to being single, no matter what your original dreams may have been? Perhaps these feelings are happening in preference to anxiety and hurt that you haven't found the relationship you are looking for yet. Perhaps what you want, deep down, is to be in a relationship.

REGRET AND FOMO

Regret is a feeling of loss or sorrow at what might have been, or wishing we could undo a previous choice we made. FOMO (or fear of missing out) is the feeling people have which spurs them into action to avoid regret. There is a famous Mark Twain saying, 'Twenty years from now you will be more disappointed by the things that you didn't do than by the ones you did.' Many single women experience FOMO, particularly the fear that they may regret not getting married and having babies. Indeed, research shows that regrets of action (doing something that turns out badly) are more intense in the short term, while regrets of inaction (failing to take a perceived opportunity) are more intense over the long term. Furthermore, the less opportunity we have to change our regretful situation, the more likely your regret can turn into rumination and depression. This is why it is so important that we are fully conscious about the big life decision that we are making, by actively choosing the things we do and don't do. Being honest about the choices we make won't guarantee that we can and will achieve all our dreams, but it will stop self-recrimination from hitting later on.

A NOTE ON NUMBING

"Numbing out" or trying to escape your feelings, through compulsive eating (bingeing), compulsive spending, excess drinking or drug taking, workaholism, even compulsive exercise or chronic TV watching are sure signs that something is up. If you think about it, no one dreams of putting on 20 kgs in a year due to late-night ice-cream binges. No one dreams of having a credit-card debt that they'll be paying off for the next seven years of their life because of shopping sprees. No one values the idea of being the world's leading expert on *Game of Thrones* (I hope!). So, whenever a behavior gets out of proportion and negatively impacts your life in some way, like these things do, it's time to stop and pay attention.

Treat these numbing behaviors like the warning light on a car's petrol tank – it's a way of our subconscious telling us that something is wrong that we are not paying attention to. Often, numbing behaviors result in dopamine spikes (the high of spending, the rush of chocolate). We are looking to feel good ... which begs the question: 'Why don't we feel good already without this fake high?'

Take the time to explore the feelings and thoughts you have just *before* you engage in the numbing. What is the painful thing you are trying to numb out from? Another way of exploring where the problem might be is asking yourself: 'If my life were perfect, what would be different?' You might not find that your numbing has to do with being single, but I've met enough single women who do numb to think it's worth a mention!

PART III

INTO THE FRAY: FROM "DESPERATE AND DATELESS" TO "SATISFIED SINGLE WOMAN"

By now we have a fair understanding of the internal processes involved in Doing Single Well. This next section is all about how to Do Single Well in our external world. Whether we choose to stay single, or we are on a mission to meet our Mr. Right, making the best lifestyle and relationship choices we can will help us feel fulfilled on our journey.

This section details the importance of having a good public relations strategy, so we can live our lives unaffected by the opinions of others. We take the time to understand our past-relationship choices and examine what happens in our brains when we fall in love, and also when we are building a longer-term relationship. For those that have been unlucky in love in the past, we explore a new perspective on choosing the right partner for you.

CHAPTER 10

HAPPILY EVER SINGLE

Whether you are temporarily single and actively looking for a relationship, or you are choosing to stay single, there are certain attitudes and lifestyle choices that will make the journey easier for you. In order to help you on your journey I have listed some things you may consider focusing on in order to Do Single Well.

FIND YOUR TRIBE

'It sounds harsh, but I just don't want to hear about breastfeeding and childcare. I can't relate to it at all! I understand that these things fill my friends' days and I do want to support them but, get a group of new mums together and you'll be up to your ears in nappy-rash talk all night!' – Jacqueline, 38 years old.

We like people who are similar to us, who share our interests, and live somewhat similar lives to us. That doesn't mean we have to ditch our old friends, but it might serve us well when we are single to find a tribe of like-minded individuals.

We all know and (mostly) understand that when a friend finds a partner and / or has a family, those people become our friend's top priority. Their lifestyle changes, and as it does, what they need from us – as well as what they can offer us – naturally changes too. This lack of reciprocal neediness can make it hard for single women to reach out and feel connected to old friends. We don't feel we can ask them over on a Sunday night to watch bad TV – they already have a partner to do that with. We don't feel we can call them up last minute for a much-needed after-work drink – they will need to get home to their kids.

One of the most common complaints single women had when I interviewed them was a lack of support – and of having to do everything themselves. Although being single had the benefit of incredible freedom, with no one to be accountable to, the downside was that no one was accountable or obligated to be there to share the burdens. Whether it's helping to change hard-to-reach light bulbs, making us chicken soup when we're sick, listening to us rehearse a work presentation, or being our "emergency contact," finding a group of friends who can support us, as we do them, can mitigate the downside that comes with the freedom of being a single woman.

Despite there not being much status given in our culture to friendships (or other non-traditional, possibly non-sexual intimate relationship models), intimacy isn't just reserved for romantic relationships. Even if the people around us aren't our "special someone," they can still help us feel that we matter; that we're worth sharing their life with.

In fact, the foundation layers of Gottman's "Sound Relationship House" can just as well be applied to friendships as to romantic connections. John and Julie Gottman found that happy couples need to know and keep updated on each other's worlds, as well as knowing how to appreciate each other in order to have a strong relationship. They called this process building "love maps" and "sharing fondness and admiration."

Knowing little things about our friends' lives and expressing appreciation for what they add to our lives also creates a strong foundation for friendship. Having a friend who remembers the major events in our history and knows who we are now – from how we take our coffee, to what our hopes, fears and dreams are – can meet intimacy needs when we don't have a partner. The best news is, close friendships like this are also less vulnerable to "growing apart."

DOING SINGLE WELL: AUDIT YOUR TRIBE

Have a think about the people that are in your life. Include everyone who you are still in contact with: life-long friends and family members, work colleagues, your church group, your tennis partner, your personal trainer, even your barista.

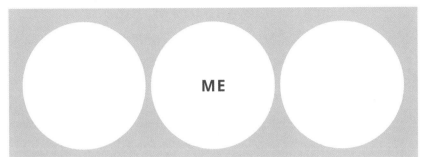

Next, I want you to place them in the circle which best describes the needs this person meets for you, which is roughly equivalent to the intimacy you have with them.

In the first circle, "Besties," I want you to put people who really know you. These are people who you could call in a crisis, who know your history, who could tell me how you take your tea and what foods you are allergic to. These people provide intimacy, companionship, and social support.

In the next circle, "Variety is the spice of life," put the people who you might not see regularly, or feel particularly close to, but still enjoy spending time with. These are the people you might invite to your next big birthday party – it could be the girl from the office that you go for after-work drinks with; the person who you see the occasional movie with, or the old friend who lives overseas that you catch up with when you travel. These people provide companionship and social support.

In the last circle, "Familiarity is comforting," put all the people you interact with who you don't really know, but can count on for a friendly smile and a little chat. This is where the barista goes, along with your dry-cleaner, your trainer, your French teacher, or bus driver. These people provide community, a sense of belonging, and trust.

As a general rule, I would like to see at least 2–4 people in the first circle; at least 4–8 people in the second circle, and at least 8 people in the outer circle. If your numbers are lacking in any circle, then have a think about what you could do to enhance your connection and establish a bigger tribe?

CASHED UP AND IN THE HOOD

Related to finding your tribe is picking a location that is conducive to connection. Single women are normal humans and therefore have innate needs to connect with others. Expecting one or two "best" friends to meet most of our needs is often unrealistic, and research shows that having a network of different types of social connections is especially good for health and wellbeing. Such a network is much easier to achieve when we live in an urban area with a bustling single community. Not only will we find that our grocery store is more likely to stock single-serve produce, we'll also find that our fitness trainer and our local barista can form part of our extended tribe, and provide the niceties of familiarity and routine.

It's not intimacy in the "love map" sense but it is nice when your coffee man knows your order and asks after you if he doesn't see you one morning. Having neighbors or flatmates that water your plants when you are away, are happy to share a meal, or are willing to look after your child while you pop out to a medical appointment can relieve some of the burden of having to do it all on your own.

Unfortunately, city-life is rarely cheap. The financial burden of doing it alone was another of the downsides most single women cited as being the cause of stress. Women in Sydney (and I would guess in most major cities) found that the cost of being single (having to pay for everything alone) and having to plan to provide for themselves when they became old or sick caused a great deal of worry.

I think there is little doubt that, in the modern world, being wealthy allows for more opportunities and less stress than being poor, whether you are single or in a relationship. Unfortunately, heteronormativity means that single women can find it financially tougher than others. Family tax cuts, savings on health insurance and holiday packages, even the scaling for bulk purchase (from the difference between single-serve yogurt and a kilo tub, to the difference in the rent on one bedroom versus three-bedroom flats) means that single women pay more. Just as in life generally, it is so much easier to Do Single Well when you are financially stable, and you don't have to worry about where your next electricity bill is coming from. The take-home here is that single women need to take control of their budgets and financial situation where possible, so they not only feel secure but they can prioritize spending money on the kinds of things that are likely to facilitate great lifestyles.

RITUALS OF CONNECTION TO SELF

The term "rituals of connection" is from the book *The Intentional Family* by Bill Dougherty (1997). In the book it refers to certain regular activities a couple can do to promote intimacy, make time for each other, and stay connected. Once again, the tools that lead to a happy married life can also support the happiness of single women. How often do you carve out space for yourself? When in your day can you stop and really pay attention to what is going on for you? How recently have you stopped to consider your hopes and dreams? I encourage you to think about scheduling some regular "me-time" to connect with your inner world, and listen to yourself as you would listen to a good friend. Some regular rituals single women have shared with me are:

- Nightly journaling
- Setting the table and having dinner "with yourself" (not in front of the TV)
- Getting your nails done, having a facial or having a massage
- Taking a bath
- Insight meditation
- Getting psychotherapy
- Taking a walk by yourself
- Sitting and having a coffee / tea by yourself with no distractions
- Going to the gym (without distractions)

Keep in mind that these activities need to promote connection to self, and a deep listening to our inner world. Pounding away on the treadmill with thoughts only of reaching a calorie target does *not* count as "good friend" behavior.

ON PURPOSE LIVING

Related to the need to connect with ourselves and spend time becoming intimate with our deep desires, Doing Single Well involves living on purpose. The life of a person who marries and has children is relatively easy with respect to finding purpose – most will say that they live for their family, or that raising their happy children has made their life meaningful. The Gottman's "sound relationship house" model for couples suggests that happy couples will make each other's dreams come true and create a shared meaning for their life.

As single women, it is up to us to make our own dreams come true and create meaning (until we find a partner, if we want one). This may be an easier job (because we don't have someone's else's dreams to accommodate) and also a harder one. For example, if you are choosing not to have children, you may have to think outside this normative box. The single women I interviewed who were not just meandering through life, and instead had something they wanted to contribute or achieve, generally felt more positive about their life. Similarly, the single women who weren't making dating their one and only priority (while not avoiding it) and still made time for other activities and connections that gave their life meaning and focus were also more satisfied.

Trimberger (2005) speaks of the importance of choosing to pursue fulfilling work, and forging connections to the next generation, when laying the foundation of a satisfying single life. I disagree that making sure your paid employment is meaningful and forging a strong connection with the young is necessary for Doing Single Well. Perhaps I'm naive in presupposing that meaning and fulfillment can be obtained outside of what you do for paid employment. Many single women might not have the luxury of time and energy to give to something meaningful in their after-work hours. However, I raise the objection for the sake of helping you think outside the box.

If you don't feel drawn to contribute something professionally and have no aspiration to mentor or care for younger people, perhaps you can explore other avenues to find purpose and fulfillment, as some of the single women I've interviewed have. To give you some examples, I've met a single woman who has developed an online course in her spare time, a couple of single women that have fostered social media communities through Facebook, Instagram, and podcasts, one that has organized the provision of necessities to third world communities, one that finds fulfillment hosting a "meet-up" group, one that lives to travel and to ski, one who volunteers to run free yoga classes in her spare time, and another that lives for her "fur babies." The limit of opportunities to find our purpose is no greater or less than the limits of our imagination. So if you haven't yet found yours, keep your eyes and ears open for inspiration.

Many great women who have achieved amazing things in their lifetime have been single – perhaps even because their time wasn't tied up in the responsibilities of a relationship and children. There are authors such as Jane Austen, Louisa May Alcott, the Bronte sisters and Harper Lee; actresses such as Mae West, Greta Garbo, Katherine Hepburn and Diane Keaton; medical visionaries such as Florence Nightingale and Clara Barton; politicians such as Queen Elizabeth I, Joan of Arc, Susan B. Anthony and Dr. Condolezza Rice; humanitarians like Mother Teresa; and artists and designers like Mary Cassatt and Coco Chanel. I would guess that in most aspirational domains, we would be able to find a single woman who has contributed amazing things, whom we could use as inspiration or as a role model.

We don't have to know our purpose right away. Nor do we have to have lofty goals and become world renowned to feel fulfilled, like the women mentioned above. Our purpose may also change over time – perhaps we will find we have a plethora of contributions to offer in different areas ...it worked for Leonardo Da Vinci! Whether grand or small, a lifetime achievement or many varied offerings, something famous or something private, your purpose is your own – and it will always suffice if it is right for you. If you have no clue where to start finding such a purpose then look back on the Values Shopping Center Exercise in Chapter 1, or the letter to yourself from the future in Chapter 9, and start brainstorming from what came up for you there.

FEEDING YOUR SKIN HUNGER

Another of the important components of Doing Single Well is to meet our own need for physical contact. This can loosely be divided into the sexual needs and the non-sexual "skin hunger" needs and both these needs can vary from individual to individual, and from year to year.

Single women will all have different libidos, and differing sexual needs, and it is likely that our libido will change over time. Many women, single or otherwise, will report not experiencing spontaneous desire, but only having their libido "turn on" after they start getting hot and heavy with a guy. Single women with this more reactive libido may never feel needy for sex if they decide to cease dating. Despite the bad press celibacy has gotten since feminism introduced an almost compulsory idea that women should desire and enjoy sex as men do, celibacy is an acceptable and enjoyable option for many single women.

At the same time, there are plenty of reasons to prioritize having a sex life, whether or not our libido is pushing us to it: some women enjoy feeling desirable, some enjoy pleasuring a partner, and some enjoy falling asleep and waking up next to someone. There is absolutely no need to give up our sex life just because we are single, particularly if we're choosing being single for life.

It's totally okay to be sexual even if we're actively dating, assuming we're not using sex to substitute for finding a partner, or hoping our casual lover will turn into Mr. Right. If you can separate sex and love, do so, and enjoy it! Whether you remain open to casual sex, find a friend-for-benefits, establish a self-love or masturbation practice, or engage a gigolo, part of Doing Single Well is exercising the freedom you have won to live life according to your terms with no accountability to anyone!

Skin hunger is the need for touch. Babies are born being able to be soothed by physical contact – it is a natural instinct for humans to pick up their babies and hold them close when they're distressed. Humans are not unique in their need for touch. Harry Harlow's 1958 study with baby monkeys showed that the babies preferred to cling to a replica mother that was made of cloth, rather than one that was made of wire – even when the "wire mummy" had the milk to feed the baby. The inference that touch and comfort was necessary to our wellbeing was also shockingly proven in studies into overcrowded Russian orphanages where adequately fed babies died because the nurses were too busy to give them affection.

Our skin is our largest sensory organ, and when it is stimulated by touch, stress-relieving and feel-good chemicals such as endorphins and oxytocin are released. Oxytocin reduces fatigue, lowers stress, promotes gratitude, regulates physical functioning, and is implicated in our bonding and attachment drives. In fact, studies have been undertaken which show that if a couple hug when they come home from work, their arguments will be reduced for the whole of the rest of the evening.

A single woman may have reduced natural opportunities to receive touch, but there are still many ways we can compensate to satisfy any skin hunger cravings. Getting a regular massage, joining a partnered dance class, even getting a pet (or sitting someone else's) can help – why not see if there's a pet sharing scheme near you? Making sure we regularly feed our skin hunger can be a good way for single women who aren't so keen on separating sex and love to go on getting some of their sensual needs met, outside of a committed relationship.

Even beyond the need for touch, there are many and varied ways to be "sensually celibate." We have been brainwashed by pornography and romance novels to equate sex with genital stimulation. However, sensuality involves all our senses. Any number of things that have nothing to do with our genitals can stimulate sexual energy and sensual passion. Trimberger (2005) gives a fantastic account of a woman who expressed her sexuality through flamenco dancing. The aliveness and passion that can be found when we engage in music, art, travel, African drumming, food, and spirituality can also be great outlets for non-genital sensual stimulation.

OPTIMIZATION: "MAKING THE MOST"

Taking a positive outlook and being grateful for the good things in our lives is helpful for everyone. However, in a culture where being single is often deemed a pitiable state, it is especially important for single women to be more aware of the benefits of being single, and make the most of them. As I mentioned in Chapter 4, single women can become very depressed if they live their lives as if they had the responsibilities and commitments of family life, without the family! There is plenty to enjoy in being single and optimizing these aspects of life will serve us well, whether we choose to stay single, or end up in a relationship.

'The best aspect, I think, is that I do whatever I want to do ... it's kind of selfish I guess, but I do love the fact that I can travel ... I can just simply buy these shoes ... If I just don't want to cook tonight, I don't ... If I just want to watch a cheesy movie I can ... If I just simply want to do a workshop the whole weekend, I will ... I don't have anyone expecting me to be there.' – Tracey, 35 years old.

Additionally, if single women put on hold aspects of their lives until they find a partner, it can make life miserable. For example, Trimberger (2005) emphasizes creating a home as an important aspect of living happily single. Whether this means buying our own place or "nesting" in a rental, by making the effort to decorate according to our tastes, creating a space that is nurturing – and that we feel we can be at home in – is an important part of life, and one that should not be the exclusive pleasure of couples. Likewise, both travel and child rearing can be enjoyed by single women, but is often put off until they meet their life partner. Doing Single Well involves taking advantage of what we can enjoy about single life, but also not sacrificing anything that we would like to experience, just because we aren't coupled.

Here's what other single women have listed as their favorite aspects of being single:

- Being able to decorate my way

- Not having to pick up after myself until I want to

- Being able to by my favorites at the grocery store

- Not having to be home at a certain time

- Being able to talk to anyone without making someone jealous

- Having time to do different things: new courses; hobbies

- Having time to read

- Quiet

- *My* music, all the time!

- Getting takeout and not being judged

- Sleeping in as long as I want

- Not having to hang out with couples

- Freedom to travel whenever

- Being able to put chocolate in the cupboard – and it still being there when I want it

- No snoring!

- No in-laws

- The seat is always down on the toilet

- I never have to watch another sport game on the TV

- I can buy as many clothes as I want, and I get the whole cupboard

The term "optimization" is used here to define the sweet spot that single women can achieve in their lifestyles. Being able to buy our favorite groceries is great, but we can optimize by also being open to trying new things so that our tastes continue to grow. Having the time to read is wonderful, but it can be optimized if we also go out and experience the joys of getting connected and being social. Spending time with friends and on hobbies is totally cool, but particularly so if we are also dating (assuming we want a partner). Think of everything in life as a continuum where both too much and too little of anything can potentially mean we miss out. Optimization of being single means really enjoying the upsides without forgoing some of the nice aspects of life that couples enjoy... Although I personally can't see any downside to always being able to enjoy having the seat down on the toilet. 😊

It makes sense that, as much as we may want a relationship, happiness doesn't naturally come just by virtue of being in one. We all know unhappy couples! And we may have had unhappy experiences of our own. Whether we are single or partnered, we have to create our own contentment, and often that requires work and balance.

As much as I recommend that single women who want a relationship make dating a priority, I will also suggest that having dating as the only top priority is a recipe for disaster. We can't 100% control how quickly things will happen for us in finding a new partner, we can only control how much effort we put in. We also need to focus on putting effort into making our existing lives fulfilling and enjoyable.

When being single feels unbearable, we can be prone to falling in love with the idea of not being single, more so than with the person who saved us from singledom! This is the definition of "settling" – that is, choosing based on fear of missing out, rather than desire for our partner. When we are content within our current circumstances, we are not so driven, and can take the time to choose a partner more wisely.

'It's about finding your own rhythm and being content with your life in the present moment, so whether you are planning on staying single, or whether you are planning on finding a partner it's about making the most of the present situation ... appreciating the freedom that you do have, while you have it, living your life the way it feels best for you at this time ... not living a life searching for something else.' – Madeline, 29 years old.

DOING SINGLE WELL ... WITH KIDS!

Firstly, if you are a single woman with children you have my deepest respect. Being a mother looks *hard*, and doing it solo must feel unrelenting. Although most of what is written in this book will apply more-or-less to you, I wanted to make special mention of the particular aspects that single moms and mummies mentioned to me when talking about Doing Single Well.

On the harder side they spoke about how difficult getting enough "me-time" was. A lack of time in general was a common theme, whether it was to put effort into dating, being social, or just keeping up with the day-to-day chores. They often talked about how they didn't have time or energy to stress over some of the finer points of housework – forget organized closets, "fussy" food and ironing! Prioritization and the need to take one step at a time became key, also saying "'no" to the people who didn't understand just how much they had on their plate.

Single mums also spoke about the financial stress of raising children, if they were doing it alone, or their ex-partners were not contributing much. Related to this, managing their feelings for, and reactions to, an ex-partner (especially in front of the kids) was an added stress that those who'd been able to completely walk away from a difficult ex, or never had a baby-daddy in the first place didn't have to deal with.

Single mums described feeling put-down by society's negative view on children growing up without a father. Some were, themselves, worried about the impact of not having a male influence on the lives of their children, and found it difficult to play the role of both nurturer and disciplinarian. They also expressed the added worry about what might happen financially, and with their children, if they became seriously ill or injured.

On the "easier" side, single mums expressed how they felt a great sense of meaning and purpose in their lives as a result of having their children. Although their children did not replace the need for adult company, they suggested that having love and family in their lives, through their children, helped mitigate loneliness. Most also said that a feeling of community was relatively easier to come by – many had made good friends with other mothers, and formed highly supportive tribes with other single mothers, which mitigated the relative lack of support that came with "doing it alone."

'I was driving home late at night in the rain with my little girl in the car and the thought popped into my head: What if our car skidded off the road and hit a tree? Would anyone notice? I know I was probably being dramatic, but that thought spurred me to get connected. I decided to check in every night with another single mum and made a conscious effort to invite friends over for a barbeque, ask a neighbor to help me move my fridge, and chat with the other mums at pre-school drop off. Slowly I realized that I didn't need a "family" in the traditional sense, I'd found a community.' – Jenna, 35 years old.

ACCEPTANCE

A lot of the ladies I've spoken to say that one of the keys to Doing Single Well is accepting where you are at in life, not looking backward with regret, or forward with worry. It's a bit like buying or renting an apartment. Once you settle on a choice, it is supremely unhelpful to keep looking at all the other apartments you could have chosen, or yearning for the apartment you had to move out of. It's far better to fix the leaky faucet, buy some new scatter cushions, and get on with the job of enjoying your new home.

Acceptance in psychology means acknowledging the reality of a situation (even if it is in some ways unpleasant) without attempting to change it, or protest against it; letting it come and go without struggling against it. Echart Tolle defines acceptance as a "this is it" response to a situation and suggests that peace, strength, and serenity are the products when you stop resisting and start accepting.

Accepting being single can be scary for some – many people equate acceptance to giving up. Acceptance is different to resignation in that it recognizes that everything in life changes, and that accepting a situation does not mean we can't work towards creating a different situation, it just means that we don't stress ourselves out in the process. For single women, this means the following:

ACCEPTANCE DO'S:

- Make it a priority to meet your own needs and actualize your dreams as a single woman

- Find people you relate to, and let people who are different to you get on with living their own lives

- Be bold and speak about your story and choices without shame

- Protect yourself from anyone who is consciously or unwittingly demeaning of your life and choices

- Optimize and enjoy everything you can enjoy about your current circumstances

- Spend time on yourself and find things that give your current circumstances meaning and color.

ACCEPTANCE DON'TS:

- Spend countless hours fretting about your future

- Ruminate on how things could have been different with your ex, or with the dates that didn't work out

- Whine about being single and be bitchy about coupled friends or "men!"

- Become maudlin and make your life into a pity party to rival Miss Haversham from *Great Expectations*

- Beat yourself up with "not good enough" gremlins

- Force yourself to download dating apps, agree to set-ups, or go on dates ... or bow in any way to societal pressure (if you prefer staying single)

- Go on pity dates, or in any way "settle" on a relationship due to fear of missing out if you want to find a relationship

- Put off life (e.g. holidays, babies, house buying) because you are single

- Avoid certain places, people or activities you would otherwise enjoy, just because you are single

"COMING OUT" AS SINGLE

'A couple of years ago there was this continual feeling that there was something missing in my life. I was in my early fifties and I was still wondering when I was going to meet a man, and resolving to try really hard to really put myself out there ... until I just went, "hey I'm so sick of thinking that I'm going to be made whole by having a man try and meet this need which is still apparently unmet." It was a story I'd been sold – that this is the way that life has to be and so I decided, "right that's it, I am not going to do this any more," and I gave myself permission to stop looking for a man. And it has been the most freeing and the most wholesome thing that I could have done for myself.' – Louise, 55 years old.

One of the highest positions of acceptance we can take in relation to being single is to "come out" and identify as single. It is completely valid to choose to stay single if a partner doesn't feature in our fantasy future. It is even a brave choice, because we will be going against the tide of what people assume to be "normal."

We don't owe anyone any explanations if we choose to stay single. Our private life is ours and we don't need to speak about it at all, to anyone, no matter who asks. However, if you can't imagine a partner in your future, you might like to consider "coming out" and identifying as single. Just as there are many benefits to coming out as homosexual for those that identify with that sexual preference, there are many benefits to coming out as single, e.g.:

- Building self-esteem and decreasing shame by being honest about yourself

- Developing closer, more genuine relationships with friends and family

- Alleviating the stress of being questioned about your relationship status in the long term

- Connecting with others who may choose to be single, and potentially building a community

- Helping to dispel myths and stereotypes by speaking about your own experience and educating others

- Being a role model for others

Coming out as single means resisting the positioning of our relationship status as being temporary, or being lacking in any way. Just like declaring a sexual identity, coming out as single means we are saying, 'This is who I am.' If you come out as single, you will need to be prepared to hold your ground firmly and resist the denial of others. The single women who I've known, who have declared their preference to remain single, have invariably been asked, 'Are you sure?' and faced comments such as: 'You'll change your mind when you meet the right person,' or 'You'll regret it when you are old and lonely.' In more extreme cases they've been called selfish, or their sexuality and their mental health has been questioned! And all by supposedly well-meaning friends and family who just can't get their heads around the idea that choosing to stay single might be the right choice for someone. You'll learn more about how to manage these reactions in the next chapter.

Interestingly, the single women I interviewed also reported the flip side: As much as they felt condescension and pressure about changing their single status, they also experienced people sharing their admiration for their lifestyle, and occasionally, even envy! This dichotomy of experience gives evidence that Doing Single Well is subjective. It's much more about your attitude (and in this case, the attitudes of those around you) than the issue of whether being single is an inherently good or a bad thing in itself.

'Some people, I think, feel sorry for me ... some of my married-with-kids friends. I think they find it quite puzzling that I enjoy being by myself. They worry that I'm missing out on the whole family thing, which I am.

But I also think that other people are envious, 'cause the grass is always greener when you're tied down with a husband and a couple of kids. The idea of being single looks quite appealing to them ... ' – Holly, 35 years old.

DOING SINGLE WELL: ARMAGEDDON ACCEPTANCE

In order to imagine what true, pure acceptance of your single status looks like, you might like to imagine that you wake up tomorrow and turn on the news to discover that there has been some kind of cataclysmic event (without the terror). Perhaps the aliens have come and spirited away all the hetero-men on the planet! There is absolutely no one to date at all, and there never will be. From now on, it's just you, doing your thing, with your tribe, making the most of the stuff you enjoy, and finding some meaning in it all somewhere. What would you be doing? Where would you spend your thinking time? What would be different to how you are living now?

Post your thoughts on Facebook @doingsinglewell

Of course, nothing remains the same in life. Even our own identity may change over time. People have been known to change their partners, their profession, their interests, their political orientation, even their sexuality! So, no matter whether you are sure that single is the right choice for you now, your feelings may change – particularly if you are a changeable sort of person.

I'm not adding my own voice to the sea of 'You'll change your mind' doubters that you'll encounter ... just asking you to give yourself permission to be human, and to change if change feels right for you. Accept and consider identifying as single now, but don't over-invest your ego in it – you might end up feeling trapped! Instead, see coming out as single as more of a signpost for you and others to understand where you are at right now.

CHAPTER 11

MANAGING THE WELL-MEANING

No matter if we are single and on the way to meeting a partner, or if we've decided to identify as, and stay single, we'll have to manage our public. You can't get away from people's opinions nowadays. Everybody is an expert, even with something as personal as how you want to live your life. So, if we are going to spend any time being single, we need to also spend some time developing our PR skills.

We can't hope to win over every doubter, but our ability to influence how people come to accept and view us as a single woman lies in how confidently we can tell our story and hold our position. The way we speak about ourselves gives subtle cues as to the amount of self-esteem or self-shame we have. If we speak about our single status with negativity or sarcasm, we are likely to elicit the same response from those we are speaking to.

In the same way that advertising sells us the best parts of a product to make it enticing, it is worth your while exploring and speaking about the best parts of living single when you are in conversation with "your public." That is not to say I want you to lie about the sucky parts and be inauthentic, but there is a time and a place (and certain people) for that kind of sharing. Pronouncing to the whole table of distant relatives at your cousin's wedding that you ate a tub of ice cream, and then cried yourself to sleep last night is *not* the best way to go to get your needs met, nor to mitigate "well-meant" criticism of your life.

So let's talk about sales ... No one would buy fizzy drinks and sodas if the adverts were all about how they made our teeth rot. Yet there are some very big brands out there that have stood the test of time because they sell themselves as happiness-making: "Open happiness." If a carbonated beverage can successfully be associated with happiness, then it should be easy for us to convince our friends and family that our current circumstances, or lifestyle choice of being single is also something that makes us happy.

DOING SINGLE WELL: SELL YOUR STORY

Compare these accounts of the same coming out story and your emotional reaction to each one. Then, have a go at writing your current circumstance or your own coming out single story.

'I'm fine on my own now, I've gotten used to my own company. And, if my ex-husband couldn't live with me then no one else is going to be able to! I'm better off doing my thing alone than putting myself through that again, especially with the amount of assholes around now. It's all too much hassle anyway, God! Getting dollied up and making small talk?! I'd rather sit home and watch the TV!'

'I got to the point where I realized I was perfectly content being on my own. I'm really enjoying my life and having my own company, and I don't see that changing. I actually wouldn't want a partner, even if someone nice came along. I love my own space and spending my time the way I want to. I love the freedom I've won since my divorce. Every night I sit in my armchair with my cup of tea, I listen to the street sounds outside and enjoy the solitude. No amount of fancy dinners or hot sex can replace the satisfaction I get from that.'

THE WELL-MEANING AND THE PLAIN MEAN

No matter how well we sell our situation, there will be individuals who refuse to let the issue of us being single lie. These are the same people who, every time they see us, ask if we've found someone yet, then shake their heads in condescending pity when we say 'no,' or tell them (again) that is not our goal. They probably have lots of assumptions about us, e.g. 'You're being avoidant,' 'You aren't doing enough to meet people,' 'You are too picky,' 'You've given up,' or 'You have low self-esteem.' Even if we are very clear and firm with our boundaries, and tell people that we don't want to speak about it, they may not listen. This is generally because the conversation isn't genuinely about enquiring after us and our wellbeing, it's about meeting some need within *them*.

These people will generally fall into one of five categories:

1. **The jilted lover:** This is the guy who thought he'd have a chance with us and is taking it personally that we choose to remain single rather than date him. As we discussed in Chapter 4, it is easier for these guys to get angry, and try to criticize, or challenge our lifestyle, than it is to feel ashamed and unlovable in the face of rejection. He meets his need to not feel rejected and "not good enough" (yes, even guys have this gremlin) by being critical and sarcastic about our being single.

2. **The egotist:** This is a person who generally thinks that they know best and challenges anyone who disagrees with them, on any issue, but in this case, on our lifestyle choice. They are usually the loud, un-empathic person who monopolizes conversations – who people try to avoid inviting to dinner parties! This person is meeting his / her need to feel superior and all-knowing by raising the issue of our relationship status.

3. **The unhappily-ever-afterist:** This is someone who is living in wedded misery and desperately trying to justify their choice, while secretly being very envious of ours. They usually have a false laugh, a tight expression, and gritted teeth when they speak of their "darling" husband and "wonderful" kiddies. You've heard of the saying "misery loves company?" This person is trying to portray us as more miserable than we are, so she can feel better about her life.

4. **The well-meaning worrier:** These are the people who genuinely care about us, but they just don't understand how a choice that has made them happy might not make us happy. In the same way that parents might pressure their children to get a further education or a job (because in their view, that is what makes for a good life), many people believe that a life cannot be complete without finding a significant other, and will worry about our choice or circumstances accordingly. This person is trying to relieve their anxiety and worry by browbeating us into seeking out a relationship.

'I've lived away from family simply because I really didn't fit their mold … I didn't want to have to be constantly asked, "Kelly, when are you going

to settle down?" My father was so concerned that I didn't have a husband and didn't have a mortgage and I didn't have security and I didn't have all the things he perceived were necessary for me to be a successful person. Then he would try to put the blame on me: "God, you are worrying me so much."' – Kelly, 50 years old.

5. **The bad conversationalist:** These are people who don't really know us, but have to speak with us at a wedding, party, networking function, etc. Characterized by their uncomfortable shuffle and the way they clutch their glass of cheap champagne, you'll find they have exactly three conversation starters: 'Do you have a partner?' 'How do you know our host?' and 'What do you do for a living?' This person is the easiest of the bunch to set boundaries with. They are feeling awkward and just trying to relieve their self-consciousness by focusing on us. You'll generally find that if you throw this person another topic, they'll happily move on to it.

No matter which category our resisters fall into, continued questions and comments that do not take our privacy, comfort, or declared preference to stay single into account can be just as frustrating and hurtful as racial or homophobic slurs. Very clear boundaries and logical consequences are the best way to deal with people who remain insensitive to us.

When it comes to assertion and boundary setting, the best way to begin is with "I statements" for example, 'I feel X …' followed by an observation 'when Y happens' and then a request 'so I'd like you to do Z.' Here are some templates you can use to develop your own assertive responses:

'I feel uncomfortable when my love-life becomes the dinner-time conversation. I'd like it if we could talk about something else.'

'I would feel so much better if we could drop this subject. I don't want to discuss my private life and need you to stop asking me if I've met anyone.'

'I understand you mean well, but as I've said before, I'm happy being single for now, and I'd appreciate it if you stopped trying to set me (or pick me) up.'

'It's a frustrating waste of both our times having this conversation over and over. Could we agree to not discuss my relationship status again?'

'I'm fed up, we've had this conversation before. If you continue to keep bringing up my relationship status, then I'm going to hang up the phone / leave.'

This last statement may seem harsh, but it is an important full-stop if our other attempts to have our boundaries respected haven't gone well. In the end, we can't choose how people will view us, no matter what we say, but we can choose whether we stay in an uncomfortable or demeaning situation.

DOING SINGLE WELL: DEVELOP YOUR OWN PERSONAL COMEBACK

Have a think about the people or situations you are most likely to get unwanted questions or commentary about because you're single. Remember, or imagine, how those scenarios usually go and take the time now to develop your own personal comeback. Remember, you'll need two or three statements of escalating intensity in case your well-meaner of choice doesn't get the hint!

We would love to hear your personal comebacks on Facebook @doingsinglewell

MANAGING THE MEDIA (BREAK OUT BOX)

I don't classify the media among the well-meaning. Preying on people's insecurities sells magazines and self-improvement products (or at least a lot of bars of misery chocolate)! So try not to believe that those perky "Seven Tips That Will Make You Irresistible" headlines are actually designed to help us. Unfortunately, these days, we are all prone to spending countless hours in a media-trance, sopping up internet articles by the dozen. I dare you to watch next time you're out and about to find someone *not* entranced with their phone! Also, because a lot of our media exposure is now internet based, it can be more difficult to tell which information we read comes from a reputable source or just sounds reputable.

For my clients with body image issues, one of the first things I ask them to do is go through their social media feeds and unfollow anyone whose posts make them feel bad about themselves. I then give them a list of "body-positive" and "Health at Every Size" organizations and individuals who produce more affirming content that they can follow. I encourage single women to do the same, even if it's just a temporary experiment to see what the effect is. Unfollow any sites or people that trigger you ... from the Bride magazines to the blogs devoted to "catching men," even the girlfriends who are constantly posting throwbacks of their wedding, or pics of the kids. Instead, follow people who are interested in what you like doing, or find and follow single woman celebrities that you admire.

THE WELL-MEANING BUT MAUDLIN

At the other end of the spectrum, we may have difficulty managing other single women. Not everyone adjusts well to being single (or reads such fabulous books as you do about how to do so 😊 and many single women have complained to me about how hard it is to keep a positive attitude when going out with their more maudlin single friends.

You know the drill. It's Friday night, you head to your local hang-out to meet up with your few remaining single friends. You order your cocktails and ask them how they're doing. One doesn't hear you because she's busy on Bumble or Tinder ... the other answers you in a distracted tone while trying to scope out if there are any hot guys in the bar. As the night wears on, hope is replaced with complaints. Stories of awful dates abound. One of your friends is feverishly spewing forth her "all men are bastards ..." BS. Another is woebegone for her empty-wombed state ... fun right?!

You may think it's the friendly thing to do to hear them both out – to nod and agree, to pat and placate, to hug and humor. You are wrong. Although kindness is key, it is better for everyone in this scenario for you to set respectful limits and empathically assert the sort of night you want to have. This may sound like:

'Ladies, tonight is our night, let's agree to have fun, and not let men or the lack of men, take it from us!'

'Hey, I know it's tough for you right now, and I think we could all do with a night off from our worries, so let's leave all that stuff behind for one night.'

THE WELL-MEANING KNOW-IT-ALLS

When we are dating, we will be bombarded by well-meaning know-it-alls. Even if we manage to avoid all the "dating expert" rulebooks on how to catch a guy, we will have friends who will want to fill in the gap. Whether these people are in a successful relationship or not they will pretend to know more about our dates than we do, and want to "help" us by telling us what he is thinking, and what we should be doing better.

I'm going to tell you a story of one of my clients to show you what I mean ...

The lady in question, let's call her Ms S (for Spectacular), was telling me about a romance she had enjoyed over Christmas time. She met her guy, let's call him Mr. EM (for Emotionally Mature) at a friend's party. They had hit it off, and so she had asked her mutual friend about him. Lo and behold, he was single but only recently out of a five-year relationship. Turns out he asked about her too, and so Ms S and Mr. EM got in touch and shared some lovely time together.

Ms S was very excited about Mr. EM. He was open and honest about his history and situation. He told her from the outset that he wasn't sure he was ready for a serious relationship so soon after his break-up. He treated her well, called when he said he would, and she felt he was a very genuine guy whom she could feel comfortable with, and know where she stood. He didn't hide his life from her, they even (albeit accidentally) ran into his mother on one of their dates, which he handled with grace and good manners. During the time they dated, she found she was able to share some of her vulnerabilities with him, and he responded sensitively. In turn, he also expressed some of his worries and "less cool" bits with her.

Unfortunately, on their last date, he told her that he had decided that he needed time alone. He told her that he really liked how, among her other good qualities, she was so caring and sensitive. She was pleased that he had picked up this more intimate knowledge of her. It showed her that he really had been engaged in getting to know her deeply. However, by the end of the conversation, she found herself still confused as to what this meant for them. So she asked if he meant that he didn't want to see her again, or if he was saying he just didn't want to be in an official "relationship." (Yay, Ms S! Way to go for being brave and reducing the ambiguity.) She told me that he thought about it deeply and seriously in front of her, taking his time before reflecting that he felt it would be best if they didn't see each other at all.

The date ended sadly but amicably. Ms S said she felt disappointed, but was also appreciative that he had been so honest, and had taken the time to treat her respectfully, right until the end. She said that, as opposed to dating in the past, she left this experience with her self-esteem intact. She had the impression that he really had been interested in her, and there was nothing that she had done "wrongly," that the relationship really had been the victim of poor timing.

Enter Know-it-all friend ...

A few days later, Ms S told her friend about what had happened. Her friend (who had never even met Mr. EM) told her that he obviously wasn't that into her. She said that if he had liked her enough it would have been the right timing. Previously secure and satisfied, Ms S then experienced a day's worth of self-doubt, anxiety, and insecurity. She spent the time running over what he had said in her head, to see where she had "missed the signs." Luckily, Ms S, confident enough in her own judgment, was able to pull herself out of this space. She told me about how she had weighed up the evidence she had about Mr. EM against the two interpretations as follows:

1. It ended because of poor timing

– he had told her from the beginning that this was a risk

– he had been open, honest, genuine, and respectful of her the whole time

– he had told her specifically what he liked and appreciated about her

– he had told her that this was why he needed to end it

– he had met her in person to end it (when others would have just let it fade away)

– She knew at least one other couple who had dated unsuccessfully at one time, only to get back together and stay together years later ... showing that perhaps timing was a genuine contributor to relationship success.

2. That he was just not that into her

– her friend thought that if he was more into her he would have made it work

– there is a common discourse in our society that any reason a relationship doesn't work boils down to there not being enough interest from one party

She also recognized that believing in her poor timing hypothesis was more helpful for her: It made her feel much better about the ending. It was not as if she could have done anything if he really hadn't been that into her anyway! Thankfully she resolved to go with her original conclusion. Why stew over an idea that just makes you feel bad, right?!

The moral to this story is that our friends are not authorities on our life and our relationships! And we are *not* authorities on theirs, so try not to be that well-meaning know-it-all yourself! Only we have anywhere near enough real data on which to make any kind of guess about the meaning of our own ambiguous dating scenarios. No friend, no rule, no book, no socially supported generality can truly shed light on our lives. Check your data ladies ... or buy a crystal ball. A hard lump of glass will shed as much light on your situation as even your most well-meaning of friends!

TRIGGER WARNINGS FOR THE WELL-MEANING

Even in the darkest and most envious hours, we know deep down that we want our friends to be happy. If they find love, have babies ... we want to be happy for them. Unfortunately, even the most well-meaning single women can be triggered when one of her friends falls in love, gets engaged, has a wedding, announces a pregnancy, or has a baby. Despite our love for our friends, their life events can be distressing for us, if these events activate an attack of our own gremlins.

'When my best friend got engaged I was thrilled for her. We had talked about how her partner was acting strangely and it was a relief to know this was why! I was happy. I told her I was happy. I even told myself I was happy ... but in reality, I wasn't. I started thinking: Why not me? Why did everything always go well for her? I spent the next week psychoanalyzing myself – why hadn't I met anyone? What was wrong with me? It didn't help that news of her engagement was everywhere! Facebook, Instagram, Snapchat ... I couldn't escape the ring pictures and the flood of congratulatory messages coming her way. I hated it and I hated myself for hating it.' – Josie, 32 years old.

If you catch yourself feeling bad about the happiness of a friend, then try following these steps:

1. Stop hating on yourself. Your feelings are perfectly normal and have nothing to do with her. You've been triggered by a situation and these feelings will pass. Criticizing yourself will just keep you stuck in your feelings and add guilt and shame to the envy you're already struggling with.

2. Have a look at what gremlins are coming up for you and try to use your strategies (outlined in earlier chapters) to overcome them. Remember: you *don't* know what the future will hold and if you want to get married or have babies, and are putting in the effort to keep dating, you are controlling everything you can control to ensure the best chance of getting what you want.

3. Reach out and say or write something nice to congratulate your friend. Buy a thoughtful gift if that is what is called for. If you don't feel you can be your best-self seeing her in person, a letter, phone call, or email is fine. Try to say something nice, and as genuine as possible – think about what you would like your friend to say to you if the situation were reversed.

4. If your friend notices something is up, or if you are very close and you feel she would understand, try being authentic with her. Tell her you want to be happy for her, but her news has triggered insecurities within you that you are struggling with. Tell her it's

not her, and ask her for her patience. You may need to take some space from her, or not be as active in the wedding / baby planning as you would like to be, but assure her that you care very much for her, you just can't show it in this way right now.

ENVY

If jealousy is the green-eyed monster that arises within us when we face the threat of losing someone or something to someone else, envy is a similar pain caused by the desire to have the advantages of someone else. Envy is always about social comparison or competition. As far as we know, envy has been experienced by all humans throughout history. In Ancient Greek mythology, Hera's envy for Aphrodite set off the Trojan war, and in the Bible, it was envy that compelled Cain to murder his brother Abel.

For envy to occur, three things need to happen. First, we must be confronted with a person who has a superior quality, achievement, or possession, in this case, a person who has met a life milestone that we want to have met. Second, we must desire that thing for ourselves (or wish the other person didn't have it so we wouldn't feel so bad) and third, we must be pained by the associated emotion.

As you can see, experiencing envy shows you (if you weren't aware before) that you have an unmet desire – you want the boyfriend / engagement / wedding / babies that the person you are envious of has. It also shows that you have gremlins. You must be feeling inferior and have "not good enough" gremlins, otherwise you wouldn't be judging yourself by comparison, and another's success wouldn't pain you.

In order to feel better after feeling envy you have two options. You could diminish your friend (by getting together with other friends and have a bitching session about her). Or you could elevate yourself. You know which one is going to turn out better for you in the long run! So next time you feel the jab of envy, try to remind yourself that although your friend is enjoying her time in the sun now, her life is not and won't be perfect. She is human, has struggled, and will struggle – just like you have and will.

Next, make a list of all your achievements. This might not mitigate the feeling of yearning for what she has, but it will go some way to fighting back the "not good enough" gremlins. And if all else fails, sometimes spoiling ourselves for the day is just the right medicine! Take a look back at the self-care list in Chapter 8 and indulge yourself ...

CHAPTER 12

THE "WHO" OF DATING

FALLING FOR YOUR PARENTS

Our brains are designed to learn, store information, and retrieve it, like a computer, with our experiences being the programming code. From the day we are born, we have experiences which we code as "love" and which condition us to unconsciously search for, and pick similar experiences when dating. We are generally drawn to people who feel like "home," namely those that have similar interpersonal styles and values as our parents ... who love like they loved.

Similarly, we develop habitual ways of relating to our parents and then relate like this with other people. Our interactions with our parents are our earliest opportunities to practice communication, and getting our needs met. These interactions help shape our view of what to expect from people. Some people relate to females like they do their mother, and males like they do their father. Heterosexual ladies can also tend to date men with traits similar to their fathers (and vice-versa for hetero guys). However, this isn't always as clear-cut, so I would advise you to be on the lookout for both of your parents' traits in your partner selection.

Falling for clones of our parents can be great news if we grew up in a nice stable home. If your mum and dad were good role models, and relatively well-balanced people, who gave you an example of how to get along with another person, and how to love unconditionally, you are set!

For the rest of us, *beware*! If your mother was critical and overbearing, you may just find yourself liking a guy who puts you down, and with whom you feel you have to walk on eggshells in order to avoid being yelled at. If you had a "busy" father who was not very emotional, you may be drawn to a man whose love has to be earned or deserved. If one of your parents liked to drink and socialize, odds are you may pick a party-boy partner.

This "bad picking" may happen in active, and in passive ways. It is very common for a single woman to actively select *out* the good guys, saying, 'Oh he's too nice' if they have had an emotionally or physically unavailable parent. The process can also be more passive, such as when a single woman is not as discerning as she could be, falling for any man who will give her attention because she has been starved of male attention as a result of an absent father.

When we are in a committed relationship, we also repeat the relationship patterns we learned. We repeat the behaviors our parents modeled for us, and how we were taught to behave towards them. The tone that is set in our parents' marriage and in our family home impacts what we consider normal or acceptable behavior. For example, if a mother stays in an abusive relationship, then her children can learn that it's okay to put up with this kind of behavior.

And if we aren't picking people similar to dear old mum and dad, we often go to the other extreme and pick someone opposite to them ... then spend the rest of our relationships resenting those differences! So, regardless of whether we are attracted to the love we found in our parents, or made a point of steering clear of that type of relationship or person, those early experiences *do* influence us.

DOING SINGLE WELL: FAMILY RULES

Thinking back to your family of origin, answer these questions about both your mother and father:

- What did they think was important in life?

- How did they show their love?

- How were your and their emotions (e.g. anger and sadness) treated in the family?

- What did they love about you?

- What did they dislike about you?

- What were their most positive qualities?

- What were their most negative qualities?

- What did intimacy look like for them?

Now, reflecting on the above questions, think back to a past relationship and see if there are any similarities or obvious opposites.

There are generally two ways we can navigate dating if we have some less-than-helpful unconscious conditioning. The first is to put less emphasis on "chemistry" when making our partner choices. This approach worked for centuries before the idea of romantic love took hold, and arranged marriages (as opposed to chemistry-fueled love matches) are still commonly practiced in many parts of the world.

There are many reasons other than bad unconscious programs to be wary of "chemistry" and falling in love: the brain in love is a brain on drugs – you'll read more about this in the next chapter. As such, it is perfectly valid to choose a partner based on other criteria and this kind of choosing does *not* mean we'll be "settling." Sure, we may not feel so magnetically drawn to our guy at the first meeting, but ... if he is a good guy who loves healthily and is patient with us (while we grow comfortable loving someone who loves differently to our parents), we *can* fall in love with him. And, the great news is that this kind of love may have more staying power than infatuation followed by drama.

Here's a story to illustrate this:

Ms O (for Once-bitten-twice-shy) came to me to make an important decision. She had two guys who wanted to be with her, and she wanted to choose correctly.

Her ex had recently come back into her life. He had broken up from his relationship and had told her that he now realized she was the one for him. She described the relationship that they had had as a "magical rollercoaster." She said that he was wild and fun, and irresponsible and free. For a "good girl" accountant like her, he added much-needed vigor to her life. She had been infatuated with him, and had also been devastated when he had ridden off into the sunset (literally – he owned a bike and had quit his job to ride around Australia).

After many months of heartbreak, Ms O picked herself up and started dating again. Eventually she met a nice man who worked in the IT department of her company. He was goofy and charming in his own way. He enjoyed his job, loved fishing on the weekends, and had the same group of friends from when he was in high school. He lived in an apartment that he owned with his small dog and, after dating for eight months, wanted her to move in with him. She said she did really love him, she just didn't get the same fizzy feeling for him that she did with her ex.

When I asked her about her parents, she looked perplexed at first. She said that her mother had met her father on holiday. He was a surf photographer and traveled around the globe photographing surf tournaments. They'd had an intense holiday fling which had resulted in an unexpected pregnancy. Her father hadn't been part of her life, excepting irregular financial contributions, and fleeting visits. When she did see him, she would be nervous and elated. He'd bring her a souvenir from an exotic location, and be full of exciting stories of tropical places and the gypsy lifestyle he led.

Over the course of our work together, Ms O worked out why she felt drawn to her ex. He sparked the same kind of anxiety / excitement that her father had. She never knew when he would be there or if he would stay ... apparently the break-up wasn't the first time he had bailed on her. When he came back to her she felt special and elated, just like the little girl she'd been who had idolized her father so much she still had every one of the trinkets he'd given her...

So the first option is that you don't have to choose based on chemistry, but what about the second option? There is a theory that those with negative childhood relationships may subconsciously seek inadequate relationships as adults to "right" the "wrongs" they experienced. Freud theorized that we continue to be attracted to the same negative experience because we want to revisit the "scene of the crime" and resolve our parent-child issues in an intimate relationship.

In order to right the wrong, we have to learn to stop being the children that we were, and stop relating in the unhelpful way we were modeled. Instead, we have to start acting like a "healthy adult." For example, in one of my own relationships, I had to learn how to tell my partner that I didn't like him being half an hour late when we made plans. My automatic habit was to pretend to be "cool" while inside feeling unimportant and resentful towards him. And yes, you guessed it … my mother is habitually a late person. We rarely complained about it as children, because we would see the fights Mum and Dad used to get into over it … essentially we learned to be "cool" about it to avoid conflict.

Being assertive, and asking for your needs to get met *will* work in any relationship. However, I give you fair warning that if you've picked a partner who is not relationship-ready, "working" may mean something different. It may "work" to filter out a bad relationship choice if your assertion results in the relationship ending (because your partner isn't willing or able to meet your needs).

It may sound easy, but if you have a lot of negative history with your parents, being authentic and assertive can be hard work at best, and re-traumatizing at worst. You will most certainly encounter some strong anxiety, guilt, and shame designed to keep you stuck in your old patterns. So, if this sounds like you, and you decide to try this route I would recommend you get the support of a counselor to help you through it.

… Ms O didn't have an easy journey in deciding on who she wanted to be with. When her ex could turn on the charm it was hard to resist him. I coached her to begin to be truly authentic with him. To tell him how he had hurt her, and to talk about the stability she desired for her life, as well as her doubts that he could provide it. Although her gremlins told her she was "boring," she wanted to have children, and she didn't want her children to have the same experience she had had.

She told me that during these conversations her ex had a range of reactions from being understanding, to poking fun at her for being too much of a "goody goody"; from being defensive and accusing her of not understanding him, to becoming sullen and sulky. It was these reactions that helped her understand the type of person he was, and to appreciate the type of man she had met in her very patient work colleague (now partner). She chose Mr. IT and they got married later that year. She has told me subsequently that she has never once regretted the choice.

DOING SINGLE WELL: THE SECRET LESSONS IN KEY EXPERIENCES

Another way to discover the rules that you might unconsciously hold and take into your dating experiences is to think back to key experiences. Key experiences are memorable moments, both good and bad, that generally have a high emotional charge. Follow this process adapted from DeAngelis (2013):

1. Make a list of the most painful and memorable experiences you had growing up, include specific events (e.g. your parents' divorce) as well as ongoing stressors (e.g. your mother's alcoholism).

2. For each memory, think about what your "take-home" was. Ask yourself: What decisions did I make about myself, others, or life, because of this experience?

3. Think about how those decisions have affected your love choices as an adult.

Example:

1. Mum and dad always fought.	2. Anger is bad, I can't show anger and I have to be good, so I don't make people mad.	3. Being overly agreeable and unassertive when dating. Not being honest about my true feelings and thoughts in case there is conflict.
1. Being overweight and teased as a teenager. Mum and Dad constantly putting me on diets.	2. It's not okay to be the way I am. I am ugly and need to change to get the love I need.	3. Putting off dating until I lose weight.

1. Mum died when I was 10 years old.	2. I have to take care of everyone. People will leave.	3. I pick men who are dependent (emotionally, financially) and when I date men who are in control of their lives and don't need me, I get anxious and don't know what they see in me.
1. Dad promised to come to my birthday but never showed up.	2. I can't trust men to do what they say. Men are unreliable.	3. I pick men who are untrustworthy and who don't do what they say, it's my "normal."

MARRIAGEABLE MEN

One of my favorite men is my teacher Michael Yapko. In his book *Depression is Contagious* (2010) he lists the qualities he thinks makes someone relationship worthy. His list (below) is a good starting point to begin to form your own ideas of what makes someone a truly relationship-ready partner. You'll notice that this list is not a checklist of status symbols (good looks, great job, university degree) nor is it about personal preferences (good sense of humor, likes the outdoors); it's all about the person's character:

1. Does he have a good sense of responsibility? Can he recognize that his actions affect others, and does he make thoughtful choices with this in mind? Can he say, 'I'm sorry?' when he gets it wrong?

2. Does he have self-awareness? Is he able to think clearly about his dreams and values and act in accordance with them? Does he do what he said he'll do?

3. What does he value? Based on how he lives his life, what can you deduce he thinks is important? Is that similar to what you value?

4. Can he accept your differences? Can he respect your boundaries and not try to change or control the things that make you, you (which are different to him)?

5. Does he have impulse control? Can he think before he acts? Can he anticipate the consequences of his words or behavior and make decisions accordingly?

6. Does he have problem-solving skills and can he adapt? Is he able to be flexible when plans change or when you give him feedback? Does he avoid problems or try to solve them?

DOING SINGLE WELL: PICKING APART HOW YOU PICK

Thinking back on your most recent dating experiences, how much of the above information did you collect?

If you didn't collect much of this information, what did you focus on instead to make your choice of whether you would continue to date your guy or not?

What might be the longer-term consequences of focusing on what you focused on, or switching to discriminating who you will continue to date based on criteria like the above?

Would you add anything to the above criteria?

How would you turn these criteria into actionable activities? i.e. What specific behaviors or stories might you look for in a date?

Post your thoughts on Facebook @doingsinglewell

DON'T BE A DELUSIONAL DATER!

'I thought he'd change his mind.'

'He said I was special.'

'But he seemed like such a sweetheart, I can't believe he did that to me!'

I couldn't count the amount of times I've heard something like this, mostly from very smart, worldly women! No matter who we are, and how much experience we have had dating, we can save ourselves a lot of time and heartache if we understand the following basic dating principles:

1. Other people are different to you

We all operate from our own frame of reference, and we tend to assume other people are more similar to us than they actually are.

However, other people do not necessarily feel the way you feel, think the way you think, or want the things you want. This is not because they are "men!" (*insert contemptuous tone here*), it's because they are *not you*.

This may sound basic, but our expectations are driven by what we each consider normal, and we are susceptible to taking these things for granted. For example, you might assume that most people your age are looking for something long term because you are. You might think that because you don't have the time to date multiple people, your date doesn't also. You might take for granted that because you would never expose your partner to sexual health risks, they wouldn't expose you to them. Or, you might assume that because you met his family he must be serious about you, because you wouldn't let just anyone meet your family.

Don't leave important expectations and boundaries unconfirmed. The conversation may begin awkwardly, but if you are really on the same page it will bring you closer together. If not ... better you know now!

2. Actions and words have to match up

Many people will tell you one thing, but their behavior will indicate another. This is not generally because they are bad people, but people can delude themselves. Sometimes what we think we want and who we think we are, is not representative of how we live our lives in reality.

What is more, this sort of delusion can be contagious! Out of a willingness to think the best of someone, and a hopefulness that the relationship will work out, you too can pretend to ignore these discrepancies! Be observant and date smart. Don't become the girlfriend of a guy who says he is ready for a relationship, when you feel you are always being put second place to work, friends, or other commitments. Or, don't keep seeing a guy who says he can't commit to a relationship just because he keeps pursuing you and seems really interested and caring towards you.

3. Know what you want and look for it early

When we begin dating, we have a window of opportunity to assess more rationally for similar values and desires. For most people, the longer they hang out with someone, the more attached they get, and the more vulnerable they are to the love drugs that will interfere with rational decision making (see Chapter 13).

I'm not saying that you have to lay it out in the first five minutes of meeting someone, but don't ignore what people say and how they treat you. Don't have sex with someone without clarifying what it means to them, and for the relationship. And, if you have been out with someone more than a few times without actually talking about what is happening, be brave! All good relationships require good communication around difficult subjects, so if you can't bring yourself to raise this issue now, it is not a good sign for the success of this relationship in the long term!

4. Let respect rule

Do not go into a relationship with the hope that you will change someone or someone's mind; that's just rude. Equally, respect yourself, and your own preferences, and don't mold yourself into what you think your date will like. Finally, assess how your date respects the areas in which you are different to him. Does he criticize you? Does he try to change you or convince you that his way is better? Can he accept the differences between you (as described in the list of qualities above)? Can you accept him or are you falling victim to settling due to your "I'm too picky" gremlins? (Take a look back at Chapter 4 for a reminder.)

Of course, we are more attracted to people who are more similar to us, but in every relationship, there will be differences. The key to a good relationship is picking someone whose differences you can live with.

Available men only!

By now you've probably gathered that I steer away from prescriptive advice and "rules." I believe everyone is an individual with their own personal history, values, and dreams, and so what is right for one person is rarely appropriate for another. I also don't believe in inauthentic dating. Following a pre-prescribed system in order to artificially enhance our attractiveness will potentially land us a partner who is not suited to us.

I do believe that, should we want a relationship, we are all worth partners who love us as we are, and make us their priority. I understand that we are in an era where many non-traditional relationship models, such as polyamory, are gaining more press. I agree that you can get a lot of satisfaction out of committed non-sexual friendships; uncommitted sexual relationships; committed non-exclusive sexual relationships, and everything in between.

However, in my clinical experience, the heteronormative model is still what most single women aspire towards. Their dabbling in other relationship models generally causes great distress and may even be seen as a form of avoidance or surrender to their "not good enough" gremlins. Perhaps this will change in the coming years when these alternative models gain more experience and wisdom, and people better learn how to "do love well" no matter what the relational structure.

For now, I promote that being secure in the feeling that, as far as your partner is concerned, you come first, is a fundamental cornerstone of secure attachment. (We'll take a closer look at this in Chapter 14.) Knowing how many single women have come to me excited about a new (unavailable) guy ... then predictably, come back broken-hearted, time and time again has led me to set the one and only rule I have for you:

If you want a partner, date available men only!

Whether it be about his situation (at this time only) or his character (who he is as a person), *you need to stop dating him if he is unavailable.*

Why? Because there are so many beautiful men out there who are available! He is not special, and you are not soulmates, or uniquely made for each other. You have a brain on drugs! (Don't worry, we'll help you deal with the effects in Chapter 13.) But if you continue to delude yourself into waiting for him, then you are wasting valuable months and years, and depriving yourself of the love that you deserve.

Oh, and before you ask, ending it means *no contact.* Measuring all the new fabulous guys you meet up against your *fantasy* of what your relationship with this unavailable man *might* become is a waste of everybody's time. No matter how many months pass, I guarantee that with permission, and assuming the connection was strong enough, he will look you up if he becomes more available for a relationship in the future. You don't need to stay in his inbox to ensure he doesn't forget how awesome you are!

So, who falls into the category of "unavailable"?

He is unavailable if:

1. **He is in a relationship or marriage – no matter how dysfunctional he says it is, or how many years they have been sleeping in separate bedrooms. If he still has regular contact with his ex around issues other than their shared children (and especially if he is still living with her), he is in a relationship. This doesn't mean that you can't date him at some point in the future but try this:**

'I really enjoy hanging out with you and I'd love to get to know you better. However, I only want to spend my time with men who are truly available. When your relationship comes to more of a conclusion, please get in touch.'

2. **He spends a lot of his time interstate or overseas:** If you can't have face-to-face, eye-to-eye, *in-person contact with him at least once or twice a week* then he is unavailable. I would go so far as to say that if he is away more than 25% of the time, he is unavailable.

We all love the excitement and fantasy of holiday romances. It is easy to assume the best about people and get caught up in delusions of how things could be when you have a partner who isn't often there in person. However, being in a partnership is all about being there through good times and bad, and relying on your partner to be there for the mundane things as well as the exciting things.

If your partner isn't there, you will probably end up relying on yourself and your social network to get your needs met. Any time you share with your partner is treated as "special" and you won't want to bring up the difficulties you are having or share true intimacy, because telling him about the "bad stuff" going on in your life could ruin the special time you have together.

Please keep in mind that if your partner is overseas / interstate or away a lot, he is *choosing something else over you*! Sure, he may be a great guy and it could be poor timing, but no matter how nice he is, or how perfect you feel he'd be if / when he moves near you or his travel schedule changes, this says he is *not* in the market for a secure relationship. And it could be that he will always prioritize other things like his career over his relationships. Try:

'I'd love the opportunity to see where this goes, but with you being overseas / interstate / traveling so much, we won't have that chance. I need someone who is willing to prioritize developing a genuine relationship with me. But please do get in contact when you move here / things change!'

3. **He puts something / someone else consistently before you:** Whether he is an alcoholic, drug addict, workaholic, overly involved with his family / kids, training for a triathlon, or just really into his dog, if he *consistently prioritizes something else over you* then he is unavailable.

Secure attachment requires a hierarchy of priorities. Partners who feel secure that they are the number one priority and are considered in the decision-making process (and have the right to veto) will generally be generous and understanding of their partner's other commitments. Think of how you would react to: 'I have to cancel our date because my teenager has just called and needs me to pick her up' in comparison to: 'I need to run something by you, I've just left to meet you at the restaurant and my teenager has called, asking me to pick her up from a party. Let's talk about what I should do.'

Give him a chance by saying: *'I feel like if it is a choice between spending time with me and (visiting your mother / hanging out with your work friends / training / walking the dog) you always choose the latter. I deserve someone who wants to be with me, not who feels that they "should" spend time with me or who treats me as the "nag," or "back-up plan." So, unless you feel that you can willingly make me a priority, I don't want to pursue this relationship.'*

If he makes excuses, says you are being unreasonable or says he will, but never does, (actions and words have to match), then you need to leave the relationship.

4. **He doesn't pursue you:** No matter how attracted you are to him, or how right you think you are for each other, if a man doesn't put in *at least 50% of the effort* to organize your catch-ups, he is unavailable. Sure, he might be socially anxious, depressed, overwhelmed with study or work. He might even express how much he is into you, and tell you how much he enjoys seeing you ... but, when men are available, and interested in someone romantically, they pursue them. So, once again actions and words have to match up. Try:

'I'd be really interested in seeing you again. How about you let me know when you're free?' Then wait to see if he walks through the door you have opened for him.

Alternatively, you might be telling yourself that if he just hangs out with you more he will become more attracted to you. In this case, you are selling yourself short. If you have anything more than friendly feelings for him, then don't torture yourself with hope when there are tons of men who would trip over themselves for the chance to date you! Why satisfy yourself with the crumbs of one man's attention when you could have all the love and attention you deserve from another?

CHAPTER 13

THE DATING DRUGS

THE BRAIN IN LOVE

'It was meant to be.'

'He is my soulmate.'

'But I love him!'

I love a good romantic fantasy ... "Twin Flames," "Soul Mates," "Mr. Right," "The ONE," and "Other Halves" are all beautiful stories! A lot of people who fall in love describe it as a transcendent, almost spiritual experience. And it is! The brain in love is a brain on drugs. The types of neurotransmitters released when we fall in love are the same, or similar to, the sort of transcendent experiences some people have on certain drugs. Falling in love is a natural high that you can thank your neurotransmitters for. Who said that neuroscience wasn't romantic!

If you have had such an experience, you'll know there is little else in the world to compare to it. Because it feels so good, we have a tendency to believe those feelings. This is called emotional reasoning (have a look again at the table in Chapter 4). We disregard reality and believe that they are "the one," they are our "soulmate," and it is "meant to be." We're convinced that we won't ever feel like this about anyone else (yes, that old man myth)! It is the combination of the intense feelings of love-highs and comedowns / withdrawals, plus these unhelpful thinking styles that make us stay hung up on someone far longer than is sensible. Falling hard for someone can unhelpfully blind us to other information that may suggest that our new "soulmate" isn't actually a good pick for us.

Another problem is when we hold out for this experience in the hope that we will feel "lightning bolts." With the right person, love can build, just as well as it can strike. Giving your date a chance to grow on you is not "settling," it is actually taking the time to make a well-informed decision ... probably one of the most important in your life. I will never encourage you to stay with someone who you don't truly love, but I do encourage you to give that love a chance to develop. What you will find if you keep an open mind is that you will either become more curious and interested in your date over time, or get more bored and switched off.

Knowing what is happening in our brains when we have "chemistry" with someone won't stop it from happening. Just as knowing what our parents taught us about love doesn't stop us from falling for people who love the same way. However, this knowledge can help de-mystify the process somewhat, and potentially give us the wisdom to be cautious of making life-altering choices based on what is essentially a natural, and temporary high.

If, after reading this chapter, you are interested in more detail in this area I'd recommend the work of my teacher Stan Tatkin, *Wired for Dating* (2016) and *Wired for Love* (2012) and Helen Fisher, *Why Him? Why Her?* (2010)

THE ADDICTION OF ROMANTIC LOVE

Romantic love is probably better viewed as an addiction, rather than an emotion. The dating brain is the addicted brain. Everything that occurs when we find ourselves "into" someone is because of the chemicals released in our brain. These chemicals change the way we feel, and we can lose our judgment. The process generally happens like this:

1. We pick up pheromones and cues about our date's immune system through scent which helps us determine whether we are suitable for one another.

2. Testosterone in men and estrogen in women is released to make you feel attracted and drawn to your date. Helen Fisher calls this the lust phase – it is different from love. Injecting men with testosterone makes them desire a potential date more, but not necessarily fall in love with them.

3. Dopamine is released to make us feel good. Dopamine is associated with motivation and goal-directed behavior, hence the drive to pursue your date. It is a short-lived, feel-good chemical which gives us a sense of joy, and a warm, expansive feeling in our chest. It increases novelty – our date seems exciting and special to us. Our world becomes brighter, we are emboldened, we feel more capable and creative, and memories are more easily made. People with addictions, or those on drugs (particularly cocaine) may struggle to experience being in love because of overuse of this dopamine addiction system.

4. Noradrenaline makes us interested. We achieve high levels of attention and energy, our thinking seems clearer, we are more aware, more awake, more focused, and more responsive. We lose the need for sleep or food. Our heart beats faster, our palms become sweaty and our pupils dilate (the "come hither" look). Sometimes, feeling increased adrenalin due to other factors can be mistaken for attraction. Dutton and Aron (1974) in their famous "rickety bridge experiment" found that more men felt attraction towards a female interviewer when she asked them questions in an anxiety-provoking environment, e.g. a rickety suspension bridge, as opposed to a calm environment. This has implications for single women who fall for "bad boys." Someone who is dangerous and treats us in ways that cause anxiety may well generate adrenalin that we may mistake for excitement and attraction.

5. Serotonin drops which leaves us obsessing over our date after we leave them. The more we obsess, the more we are likely to seek them out again. There is some evidence to suggest that people on antidepressants (Selective Serotonin Reuptake Inhibitors) struggle to fall in love as they don't experience the serotonin drop that causes them to crave contact with their date, making them think he's not the one.

DOING SINGLE WELL: RE-LIVE YOUR DOPAMINE RUSH

Want to know what a dopamine rush feels like? Close your eyes, take a few deep breaths, relax ...

Now think about a happy memory. It might have been having fun with someone you love, enjoying a tasty food, fantasizing about your celebrity crush, the day you won that prize, or anything else that leaves you feeling warm and fuzzy. Get lost in the details. Was it day or night? What was the air temperature like? Was there a breeze? What was around you? Fill in the colors, shapes, sounds, and smells. If you started smiling, it's because your recollection triggered a dopamine rush in your brain!

Post a photo of a dopamine moment on Instagram #doingsinglewell or write about what it felt like to you on Facebook @doingsinglewell

YOUR CHEMICAL SIGNATURE ...

Helen Fisher proposes that the neurotransmitters described above are present in different proportions in different people. The proportion of each chemical in your body determines what types of dates you are likely to fall for. In this way, she suggests a "nature" (i.e. biological) rather than a "nurture" (i.e. learning from your family of origin) explanation for the attraction or "chemistry." In reality, given that all our experiences affect our brain chemicals and vice-versa, I suggest that falling in love comes down to both love drugs *and* parental programming.

According to her model, there are four main personality types based on the levels of the production of four chemicals in your system: dopamine, serotonin, testosterone, and estrogen:

1. **Builders** – High in serotonin. Cautious individuals who tend to follow traditions and value persistence. They are relaxed, social, conscientious, steady, and family and community oriented. They tend to fall for other builders.

2. **Directors** – High in testosterone. Analytical personalities who enjoy making decisions. They like competition, can be highly ambitious, and can have a tendency towards aggression. They tend to have good self-confidence, are straightforward, tough-minded, focused, pragmatic, and value logic over emotions. They can have excellent spatial, musical, and athletic skills. They tend to fall for negotiators.

3. **Explorers** – High in dopamine. Risk takers who are impulsive, adventurous, sensation-seeking, and creative. They can be highly motivated, focused, energetic, and goal oriented. They can also be prone to boredom and tend to seek a playmate in a partner. They tend to fall for other explorers.

4. **Negotiators** – High in estrogen. Intuitive, idealistic, and empathic individuals who are more selfless than the other three types. They think abstractly and flexibly, they have a vivid imagination, and tend to seek a soulmate in a partner. They are more introspective and emotionally expressive. They tend to fall for directors.

You might relate to features of several, if not all of these types, but most people are dominant in one or two. If you want to find out what your chemical profile is, you can take Dr. Fisher's free test online: https://theanatomyoflove.com/relationship-quizzes/helen-fishers-personality-test/.

Dr. Fisher poses that your chemical profile influences who you are likely to have chemistry with, but she does say you can fall in love, and have successful relationships with any type. She details all the combinations on her website with a horoscope-like strengths and weaknesses list for each paring.

DOING "CHEMISTRY" WELL

After the age of 25 (when our brains are fully developed) we can trust our automatic brain to select a person based on what is familiar and attractive to us. It isn't a conscious decision, we just "feel" it. Selecting based on this chemistry might mean we can meet someone who ticks all the boxes but then find that we are just not that into them. It is also the reason why we find ourselves attracted to a guy who we know isn't a good pick (or just like our dad in all the wrong ways).

Because the chemicals behind the feeling of love alter our judgment, as can our family-of-origin experiences, doing "chemistry" well means choosing a partner with both our emotional and our rational brain. Our family or origin and our chemical signature might influence our feelings, but our reason (if we can access it) is more resilient. Feel it … but also think about whether the person can give you what you want.

One of the best ways to make sure our altered mind makes the right choice is to get feedback from trusted friends and family after hanging out with us and our new partner. Because they know us well, and their brains won't be addled with love drugs, they'll be in a far safer position to tell us what's what. No one wants to hear that the guy they brought to dinner is a sanctimonious turd who, to anyone other than you, is more groan-worthy than great. But before we turn diva, we need to remember that divorce is both a hassle and expensive … maybe our buddies are actually trying to look after us? And if our besties aren't so brave as to butt in and tell us what they think, we need to ask them!

'It was only after we broke up that my best friend told me that she'd never liked my partner. And she wasn't just saying it to make me feel better! She recounted how horrified she had been the first time I'd brought him to lunch. She remembered how rudely he'd treated the waiters and how he was constantly on his phone … She said that I became quiet around him and that he would speak over me.' – Alice, 31 years old.

DOING SINGLE WELL: THE FRIENDSHIP FEEDBACK TEST

Have you ever had friends tell you that they hadn't liked one of your exes (and not just out of break-up sympathy)? Do you have friends who know you well enough to see how you are with a new person and say whether or not they're good for you? Try to pick friends and family who have known you a long time and who themselves have had good, stable relationships. Next time you introduce them to a new date, pull them aside afterwards and ask them questions like:

- How would you describe my new partner?

- What did you notice about us together?

- Do you think I am different around him? How?

- Do you think we are a good match?

Post your stories on Facebook @doingsinglewell

ADVICE FOR THE ADDICTED

The problem with falling in love comes when we are "hooked" on someone and that someone is not "hooked" on us. Or, they are "hooked" but are unavailable or unsuitable for a relationship.

The irony of love-addiction is that we are actually *more* likely to have an addiction problem to someone who is not 100% there for us while we are dating. A guy who is responsive and reliable is not as likely to elicit as much adrenalin / anxiety as a guy who is inconsistent. Similarly, the cravings / serotonin drop won't be as strong with a guy who is available and consistent. This quirk of human chemistry is often misappropriated by dating rulebooks (for both men and women) which advise "playing it cool" and "making him / her work for it." You can read more about what I think about *that* in Chapter 14!

A guy's ambivalence gives us what is called "intermittent reinforcement." When we get what we want unpredictably and only part of the time, we tend to stay hopeful and addicted for longer than if we had previously gotten what we wanted every time. Think about a slot machine: the slot machine pays out only occasionally, yet gamblers will keep feeding money into it for a long time in the hope it will pay out again. If the slot machine was set to pay every time, and then stopped paying all of a sudden, the gamblers who had previously been using it would give up more quickly. Think about this next time you go to initiate that next text to your only-sometimes-responsive guy!

ANTI-ADDICTION PLAN

If you find yourself unhealthily addicted to someone who is not into you, or not available for a relationship, try to eliminate all contact for the time being. Even if he does respond, having another "hit" of your favorite drug will just lead to the same old comedown and withdrawal the next day / week.

When you get the urge to look him up or contact him:

1. Have a list ready to remind yourself of all the reasons the relationship *didn't* work out or what you *didn't* like about him

while you were dating, and another list of all the things you are looking for in a relationship.

2. Remind yourself that in these situations *decisions should be made on the outcomes that you want, rather than how you feel* (because your brain is on drugs at the moment ... see point 4).

4. Act compassionately and lovingly towards yourself. Be gentle, don't get mad with your urges or your feelings, they are natural. Your brain is just in withdrawal and the feelings will pass.

5. Get distracted. Call a friend, watch a movie, go for a run ... the busier you get at this time, the less you'll notice the uncomfortable feelings of withdrawal, and the less you'll be prone to giving into the urge for contact.

You'll know you are over it when you can bump into him without feeling much, and you don't have the urge to contact him afterwards. This often happens when you are in love with someone else. However, it can also happen if enough time has passed that you are no longer hopeful things will work out between you, and you stop viewing anything he does as a genuine sign that things could be rekindled.

REAL LOVE IS ACTIONS

The secret that all long-term happily committed couples know, that the rest of us need to discover is this: the movies lie! We've all seen that peak moment of any romantic movie. The couple come together finally, the music swells, the rest of the scene fades away, and the camera narrows in on them staring into each other's eyes, exchanging earnest declarations, and passionately kissing. This is sold to us time and time again as "love" so we can be forgiven for chasing this feeling and this experience when we are dating. But of course, the movies rarely dwell on what happens after the couple declare their impassioned "I love you's." Check out Dina Goldstein's series on Fallen Princesses for a few alternative ideas!

In reality, the emotion of love, like any other feeling, will come and go. We may feel a great deal of love staring at our beloved over a dinner table one night, and then wake up decidedly out-of-sorts and definitely not feeling the love the next morning. I've seen many single women get confused and despairing about this, searching for the feeling of love, and not wanting to "settle" but having countless bad experiences and heartbreak. Be careful of "chemistry" and the feelings of infatuation and romantic love. Yes, it is magnificent, and a worthwhile experience if we can have it. But no, it is not the be-all-and-end-all of what we should be looking for in love. It is only one component of it.

To recap, attraction goes beyond the first glance, superficial, "hot-or-not" impression. Research has shown that attraction has much more to do with who you are as a person, and how well you can relate to your date (for more, see Chapter 7). Having chemistry with someone and "falling in love" has got to do with your unconscious ideas about love, learned from your family of origin (see Chapter 12) and your neurotransmitters (see above). Staying in love, what I term "real love," has to do with actions. This is why it might be better to judge your date based on their character (see Chapter 12) rather than just how you feel.

It is *normal* for long-term couples to "fall out of love" and to stop feeling the fireworks they used to feel. Long-term couples have to form habits of looking for, remembering, and communicating the reasons why they love each other so that they can continue to experience these temporary warm and loving feelings towards their partner. The Gottmans say these habits of expressing "fondness and admiration" and of "turning towards" what our partner says and does are important components for making love last. Similarly, continually updating our "love maps" of our partner's internal world, through talking with our partner, and developing "rituals of connection" to spend quality time with them are seen as important actions.

In his now famous book, *The Five Love Languages* (1995), Gary Chapman defines five categories of actions that people express and experience love from: tokens (giving and receiving gifts); time (spending quality time together); talk (words of affirmation); tasks (acts of service) and touch (sexual and non-sexual affectionate touch).

No matter what model we are using, it is clear that love isn't just a temporary feeling. Real lasting love is more associated with loving actions. The wake-up cup of tea brought to bed; the thoughtful gift; the genuinely interested 'How are you?'s are actually what love is.

Due to the neurochemicals we have described, these loving actions can happen more naturally and automatically when we are first dating, and feeling like we are falling in love. As such, we can be forgiven for thinking that these actions are the consequences or end result of feeling "in love." Instead they are the essential ingredients or precursors of real love in the long term. And we'll talk more about these actions and the attachment chemicals in the next chapter …

CHAPTER 14

ONCE THE HONEYMOON IS OVER

It is thought that humans are designed to attach to each other because human babies are born relatively vulnerable and need their parents' protection. Unlike a foal, human babies can't walk and feed themselves when they are born. Unlike a nest of baby snakes, our parents generally only have one baby at a time, and so stick around to ensure their survival.

Attachment is the bond that keeps people together past the initial spark of attraction, or once the "chemistry" has worn off. Research says that the "limerence" period of new, sparkly, amazing, dopamine-fueled love lasts for about 12–18 months in most couples. Once these feelings wear off, we have two main chemicals that make us attached and keep us together: oxytocin and vasopressin.

Oxytocin is known as the cuddle hormone; it is released during cuddles, childbirth, breastfeeding, and during orgasm in both men and women, and it is thought to make people feel closer and more caring towards each other. Animal studies have shown that if you block oxytocin in rats they reject their young, whereas if you give it to female rats who've never had sex they begin to fawn over, nuzzle and protect another female's pups as if they were their own.

Vasopressin is also released after sex. It is thought to have a role in long-term pair-bonding after studies on the prairie vole. Prairie voles form fairly stable pair-bonds usually (they also tend to have a lot more sex than they need to for reproduction)! When vasopressin was suppressed in male prairie voles, the bond with their partner deteriorated and they stopped protecting their partner from new suitors.

Just like different people have "chemistry" for different types, different people have different styles of attachment. An attachment style is a pattern of behavior that was most likely to get our needs met in our family environments. That is not to say different attachment styles don't have different nervous systems and chemical profiles, they do. "Nature" and "nurture" are actually hard to tease apart when it comes to nervous systems and early childhood experiences. Our "nature" affects how our parents "nurture" us, and the "nurturance" we receive makes fundamental changes in how our brain is wired, producing our "nature."

As we discussed in Chapter 12, how our parents related to us, and each other, has a big subconscious impact on how we learn to relate to others. We won't be consciously choosing the feelings, thoughts, and reactions we have in relation to a loved one – they will bubble up quickly and spontaneously. We can, however, educate ourselves about our habits and tendencies, and learn to respond differently to the thoughts and feelings that occur for us should our automatic responses be unhelpful.

There are plenty of different models of adult attachment styles. I'm going to use the one that Stan Tatkin uses in his books, as I think it is a practical way to think about these things. In his model, there are three main styles, but, as with most models, you may find you have elements of them all.

SECURE ATTACHMENT AKA "ANCHORS"

About half of all people are primarily "anchors." Anchors were raised with at least one parent who put their child's needs before their own. Anchors were appropriately soothed and comforted as children, but they were also encouraged to be independent, and to cooperate with other family members. In anchor families the emphasis was on relationships, so if you are an anchor, you would have experienced justice, fairness, quick conflict resolution, and sensitivity in your family.

As such, anchors grow up to be well-adjusted adults, who can get along with anyone, and have positive views of themselves, their partners, and their relationships. Anchors can talk about themselves and their feelings and can read themselves and others well. They are flexible and resilient.

Anchors have an easy time transitioning from alone-time to "us-time," and they feel comfortable with intimacy and with independence, balancing the two. They don't fear being smothered or abandoned and this makes it easy for them to commit and be emotionally available in relationships. They prefer to be with their partner but don't cling and, upon separation, they think about their partner fondly.

Important note: everyone *looks* like an anchor early on in dating, but attachment patterns only generally come out once you really start to like someone and the relationship has become more "permanent."

AVOIDANT ATTACHMENT AKA "ISLANDS"

About 25% of the population are primarily "islands." Islands had parents who stressed performance, intelligence, talents, or appearance, and discouraged any neediness. At least one parent was probably emotionally distant, and they may have used money to buy their children's love. Because the island's parents were more focused on themselves than their children, the island learns to rely on him or herself, meaning they need a great deal of space in relationships. Without that space, islands may feel smothered and controlled by their partners.

Islands feel more relaxed when they have alone-time and, it can take time for them to switch from alone-time to being with people, as if they get into a trance-like state of focus when entertaining themselves. They are often very logical, practical, and detail oriented, but often don't understand, or have many words to talk about themselves and their feelings – and can be prone to shame and guardedness as a result. They value self-sufficiency and being "low maintenance," and they seem not to mind doing things separately, or being separated from their partner.

ANXIOUS AMBIVALENT ATTACHMENT AKA "WAVES"

"Waves" also make up 25% of the population. Waves had parents who were emotionally inconsistent, here one minute and gone the next (emotionally or physically). This results in waves growing up to fear abandonment above all else. Children of addicts are often waves. Waves can be needy in relationships – requiring constant validation that their partner loves them and is there for them.

They tend to be less trusting, and have less positive views about themselves and their partners. They may exhibit high levels of emotions and are prone to worry and impulsiveness in their relationships. They like to talk through things (sometimes excessively) and can worry that they are "too much" in a relationship. Because of their abandonment fears, separations are difficult for waves, and they can display angry and rejecting behaviors upon reunion.

DOING "ATTACHMENT" WELL

Although everyone wants to be an anchor, it is important to realize that none of these attachment styles are defects. Single women with all three attachment styles can form secure relationships when they meet a healthy partner, and when they have developed self-awareness. No matter which attachment style you identify with, don't beat yourself up. Use the information to shed some light on past relationships that didn't work, and to be forewarned and forearmed about what you might expect to bubble up for you after the first few dates with the next new guy you are into. Remember that although most people can act "secure" during the early stages of dating, you may find that your attachment tendencies (and his!) begin to show as things progress.

SINGLE WOMAN WAVES

Some of my wave single women will find themselves on an emotional rollercoaster when dating, and come to me with high anxiety. They often know they are being unreasonable and hate the way they are acting towards their guy, but can't seem to stop themselves. Here's a story to show you what I mean. Hopefully you'll be able to see both Ms W's wave tendencies, and her partner's island ones:

Ms W (for Wave) came to therapy because she desperately wanted a partner and family, but found that she couldn't meet the right man. She despaired that there was something wrong with her and that she was "unlovable" because she was so "high maintenance."

She described with embarrassment how, in her last relationship she would be ultra-sensitive to being ignored. Her partner had been a busy business owner, but when he didn't call her during the day, return a text she wrote promptly, or if he wrote back too briefly for her liking, she would be irate! 'It felt like I wasn't a priority, I'd get so mad because I'd see him online and knew that he could see I was online too, but he couldn't even be bothered to say, "Hey!" I knew I was being unreasonable, but I couldn't stop the feelings.'

She also spoke about how she grew agitated when he came to her house. All he wanted to do was snuggle on the couch and watch TV, but she wanted to talk! She said that even when they did talk he'd often pull out his phone and begin playing on it, while they were speaking. She said she found it hard to get to know him, and felt he wasn't really interested in asking deep questions of her. When walking he'd often walk ahead of her, unaware of how alone this made her feel, and when they were out socially, he'd go off and speak to his friends and leave her to fend for herself. She felt unfulfilled and yearned for more closeness, even though she could tell he was trying.

All the difficulties in their relationship made Ms W anxious. She was worried she was wasting time with him, and was constantly anxious about whether he would pay attention to her and make her feel good, or if he'd trigger her anger again and they'd get into a fight. She broke up and got back together with him again and again. She hated the rollercoaster of anxiety and anger she was on, and eventually ended the relationship out of exhaustion.

SINGLE WOMAN ISLANDS

Although guys generally show higher avoidance than anxiety, ladies can be islands too. My island single women will often present with less motivation and low energy when talking about dating. They tend to prioritize other things, and deep down, feel inadequate when it comes to relationships. Here is a story to show you what I mean:

Ms I (for Island) had been ambivalent about getting into a relationship for many years. On the one hand she did think she wanted one, on the other hand it seemed like so much hard work.

She lived with a flatmate who was an air hostess and rarely home, but she didn't mind that as she liked her own company. She confessed to me shamefully that she often fibbed and told her friends that she was busy when they asked her out, just so she could have a night in. She'd screen her calls, so she could spend her time reading and watching TV. She had a very busy and important job in IT and was one of her company's star performers, but it meant that she had little juice left in the tank for others, and often found some people in her life a burden.

When she did meet new people, she felt like she was performing. She didn't know what to say when people asked her to talk about herself and described to me how she'd learned early on to entertain people with funny stories, impress them with her accomplishments, or focus the conversation on the others: 'I got really good at asking the questions … people love talking about themselves and it helped the conversation flow.'

Ms I had been on many dates, and had even had some short-term relationships, but things rarely seemed to progress. The guys who were "constantly" messaging, or calling (once a day) annoyed her – 'I don't have anything different to say from yesterday! Nothing's happened!' And she hated the ones who got "handsy" – 'I just don't see why people have to be all over each other.' On the other hand, when she met guys with a similar schedule to her, things seemed to fizzle out.

Doing "attachment" well involves starting to understand your attachment patterns and predispositions. Once you know your tendencies, the aim is not to try to change them, just bring about awareness of them with the guy you are seeing so that they don't interfere and aren't misinterpreted. For example, Ms W had to learn to say things like: 'I know there are people who need to get hold of you, but I like to feel important, and to feel that you want to spend time with me. I don't get that when you are always on your phone. Can we agree to put our phones away when you come to my place?' Ms I had to learn to say things like: 'I like you a lot, but I'm not a very touchy-feely person. If you feel me stiffen when you hug me, it's just because it takes a while for me to get comfortable.' You can read more about dating with this type of authenticity and self-acceptance in the next chapter!

PART IV
A FRESH APPROACH TO DATING

In this section, we will explore how following dating rules and "playing it cool" contributes to the bad experiences single women have. The fresh approach of authentic dating is detailed as an alternative to help single women maintain their self-esteem, practice the essential relationship skills of assertion and boundary setting, and minimize broken hearts and bad dating experiences. We look at how to stay authentic while internet dating, and give an authentic approach to dealing with a heartbreak.

CHAPTER 15

RULES VERSUS AUTHENTICITY

COOL CATS

There is a lot of advice out there for both men and women to play it cool while dating. Don't be too keen. Don't make the first move. Don't say 'I love you' first. Keep them guessing. This advice has some scientific basis, but it misses out on humanity!

When we play it cool with someone who is interested in us, we are essentially pretending we are unavailable or relatively uninterested in them. This will increase their anxiety, and also their relief when we finally throw them some attention. As we spoke about in Chapter 13, this intermittent reinforcement is one of the ways to get someone very addicted to you fast. But why would you want that?

When you think about it, a single woman who plays it cool must be doing so because she doesn't believe her own natural charms are enough to keep someone interested. Instead of being real and having genuine responses, she plays her dates in a game of cat and mouse. She is the cool cat, and the men she dates are the pitiful mice. It's an entertaining power dynamic. Who doesn't get a thrill when they have someone chasing them? But is that really how we want to run our relationships? I propose that having unequal power (and playing games) is not the strongest foundation to build a life-long match on!

What is more, single women who play it cool are also protecting themselves from vulnerability. Ice queens never put their heart on the line to try to protect themselves from getting hurt. They feel safer because if things go badly they haven't opened themselves up too much. However, that does not mean that if it doesn't work out, they don't feel equal amounts of disappointment, compared with someone who has been more open. Maintaining one's pride or saving face is generally a cold comfort, given that the feelings might be there whether you put your heart on the line or not!

Furthermore, without vulnerability there can be no real connection or intimacy ... and why do we date if not to develop intimacy?! As the old saying goes, 'It is better to have loved and lost than never to have loved at all.'

Think about a role reversal: How would you feel if you found out that your date was playing it cool with you to try to ensure your interest in him. Wouldn't you feel a bit ... well ... played? And what happens to you when someone is self-consciously being cool with you? Does it make you feel secure, confident, hopeful, loving? Or anxious, preoccupied, and frustrated, not to mention worried that the relationship is hard work and ultimately fragile?

It is for this reason that anchor men don't respond particularly well to playing it cool. A man who has a strong sense of what mutuality is in a relationship won't take kindly to being played with, and is just as likely to call you out on your games as he is to move on to someone more emotionally mature who knows what she wants.

> **Showing a guy that you are interested in him is not shameful, or a weakness.**

At worst, he will be flattered, but not reciprocate – this is rarely a life-changing embarrassment. Just think about how you would react if someone revealed unwanted interest in you? You are barely going to think about it in a week, let alone a month, or a year from the awkward conversation. Yet, if you are interested in him, think of how encouraging it would be to know that he is keen too! So, dear single women, remember: nothing ventured, nothing gained!

RULES VERSUS AUTHENTICITY

To recap, our definition of authenticity is 'the daily practice of letting go of who we think we are supposed to be and embracing who we are' (Brené Brown, *The Gifts of Imperfection*, 2010, p.50). As such, being authentic is a key skill to develop when it comes to dating. It can be so tempting to be what we think a new date wants us to be, or to follow some set of prescribed rules some "expert" gives us to keep ourselves safe. But when we do this, we are doing both ourselves and our dates a disservice. Why waste time wearing a mask or performing a role? If you end up together, he'll get to see the real you sooner or later!

There's no doubt about it, rejection stings. But it's far better to be rejected for who we are early, than to be accepted for who we are not. No one wants to be trapped playing a role, or invite criticism when we start to show our true selves. Our society pushes perfectionism onto us all – we need to have the perfect body, the perfect job, the perfect lives, and be the perfect partner. The issue is that when it comes to dating "perfect" is a subjective term. One guy might want a girly girl who bakes cookies and darns his socks. (Seriously?! Just buy another pair!) Another guy might love a girl who can rough it camping, and impale worms on to fishing hooks ... clichés aside, you get my drift, right?!

Being authentic is a brave choice. It is brave because it flies in the face of our natural fear of criticism and rejection. You can't be courageous without having fear. As daters, we fear that if we show up as we truly are – saying, doing, and feeling the real things that are going on within us, without augmenting or censoring ourselves in any way, our dates might not be interested in us. When we are authentic, we are choosing this discomfort now over discontentment later. It might be uncomfortable being vulnerable and honest about ourselves, but it is eventually more satisfying than the discontentment of a poorly matched or inauthentic relationship.

Being authentic is also a risky choice. Just because we have courage doesn't mean we will "succeed" if by that we mean getting the guy. This is why dating rulebooks are bad. They prey on single women's low self-esteem and fear of not being good enough, or of getting it wrong, (thank you, gremlins)! The books go on to tell us they can minimize the ambiguity of dating by giving us rules that will lead to "success" at catching guys. These rules purport to make "known" the "unknowable" by giving answers that can't possibly be true 100% of the time to questions such as: "How do I make him like me?" "How do I get him to commit?" But that only gives a false sense of safety and security. The dating world seems easier to navigate with some "expert's" rules in our back pocket!

Rulebooks also act as a vulnerability shield. If we get rejected, we can claim it wasn't really about us – the rules just didn't work with this guy. Or, as the rulebooks would have you think, this guy was obviously unworthy. However, in exchange for safety and protection from vulnerability, we lose the potential for intimacy. We can't have intimacy without deep knowledge of someone else, warts and all. When we play by rules we are playing a role of "temptress," "perfect girlfriend," or "cool" (or someone's idea of those roles anyway)! And in the process, we are stamping down on all our natural instincts, needs, and feelings.

Instead, the crazy, risky, scary, amazing, and inspiring journey that is being truly authentic has these three components:

1. **Knowing yourself** – knowing your preferences, values, and dreams. Knowing also your gremlins, man myths, and any unhelpful relationship rules and attachment patterns you developed growing up and accepting yourself with this imperfection.

2. **Owning your stuff** – taking responsibility for your contribution compassionately. That means no beating yourself up, and no blaming him. Being kind. Being real. Telling him honestly what is happening for you, even if it feels vulnerable.

3. **Setting boundaries** – being aware of your feelings and saying nice 'No's to things that don't work for you, even if it means that you might lose the relationship.

To show you the difference, I've put a few of the most famous dating "rules" against an authenticity approach. As you'll see, there is a potentially frustrating level of ambiguity about the authenticity approach, but I hope you'll also be able to see the relative freedom and mutual respect that is inherent in it too!

RULE / AUTHENTICITY

Take care of yourself! Be beautiful, fit, feminine. Smell good.	Invest in your self-care for *you*. Make yourself feel good, and wear what you like and feel good in. If you like certain scents, wear them, if not, don't. Let how you care for yourself be a part of your personal self-expression and self-love.
Make him approach you. Don't be a hunter.	If you see someone you like the look of, make eye contact and smile – if you can be brave enough to go over and chat, then you go girl! Go after what you want. As in life, so in dating, it's better to have tried and failed than to not have tried at all.
Never be offended.	If a man is critical of you, clarify what he meant (to ensure you aren't misinterpreting), then set an assertive boundary. e.g. 'I don't appreciate you calling me "blonde" in that tone.' You deserve to be treated well!
Don't chase and don't wait.	If you are interested in a man, show it. If he is not interested back, not available, not putting in equal effort, or has a tendency to leave you hanging, then set an assertive boundary and move on. e.g. 'I'd be interested in taking this further, but I need to be with someone who can be more consistent in responding to me. If your circumstances change, look me up.'
Don't call him back immediately, end a call after 15 mins.	If you are delighted by his call, then pick up, and tell him how happy you are that he called! If you are enjoying chatting to him, and have the time, not only keep chatting, but tell him how much you are enjoying it!

Wait at least four hours to respond to texts, write fewer words than he does, never double text.	Hopefully you will be out, living a great life and not on your phone 24/7 … Respond when you notice the text, or when you next have the time to give it the response it deserves. Give whatever response it is within you to give. Triple text if you want to (or pick up the phone and call him if there is a lot you want to say) so long as you are owning your stuff and not disrespecting his boundaries. See Chapter 17.
Don't reveal too much.	Tell him about yourself, ask him to tell you about himself. Gradually exchange deeper degrees of intimacy and vulnerability. Nothing about you is shameful, or needs to be kept secret. If he wants mystery he should date Agatha Christie.
Be supportive and sympathetic but don't ask for sympathy.	Be kind if he needs sympathy, but if he is monopolizing the conversation, gently tell him there are things you'd like to talk about too. If it is you who needs sympathy and care, ask him to give it to you. We all have emotional needs and we definitely want a partner who can meet them! See it as a good screening procedure!
Be happy, never sad or bossy.	Be yourself with the full spectrum of your human emotions – just own them and don't blame him for them.
Judge him by the type of gifts he gives you.	Appreciate his gifts and, if they don't suit you, or they suggest that he doesn't know you very well, gently correct him. 'I love that you thought of me and want to share this with me, but I'm not such a fan of rock concerts, they give me migraines. I wonder if you could take a friend and we'll do something else together?'

Don't see him more than 2–3 times per week.	Lead a fulfilling life, full of things you enjoy, in addition to dating. Don't put your life on hold to see him, but also make sure that dating is a priority if you want to be in a relationship.
Only casual kissing on the first date. Don't have sex, and when you start having sex with him, don't then withhold sex from him in the future.	Be aware of yourself and your feelings. Only become sexual when you are feeling safe and curious about having sex with him, not because you feel you "should" or he expects it. As a general rule, if you are feeling comfortable enough with him that you know you could ask him to stop half-way into the sexual act and he'd respond supportively then you are intimate enough to have sex. Respect yourself and your ever-changing sexual needs and desires, and communicate them accordingly.
Be busy and don't explain.	Be available. Show him the respect you would like to be shown by returning his calls, responding in a timely fashion, etc. You don't have to explain or justify yourself, but if the situation were reversed and you would appreciate an explanation, treat him with equal kindness.
Don't talk about him to others.	Share your feelings and thoughts about him with others as you usually would with anything happening in your life. Self-disclosure will bring your friends closer, and your friends can be a good resource in helping you determine if he is good for you when they meet him.
Don't talk about the future.	Talk about your hopes and dreams. If you want to get married and have a family, there is no shame in that – talk about it! Likewise, if you want to get serious with him, it's a compliment!

Don't criticize his life.	Criticism is rude, don't accept it or give it. Be honest. If you don't like something about his life or choices say so with kindness. Eg. 'I can understand that you like them, but I'm not a huge fan of cigarettes and I don't like the smell.'
The relationship ration should be: him 70%, you 30%.	If you are both interested in a relationship, the effort you put in should be 50/50. Being available creates mutual security and we want a secure-functioning relationship.
Make him make up excuses to see you.	Be available and let him know he is welcome to ask you out if he wants to see you. Similarly, ask him out if you want to see him. Treat him with the same care and respect as you would a close friend. Men are people too!
Never ever agree to a date that is less than 24 hours away.	Keep a fulfilling social life; don't change your plans to be with a guy. But if you have nothing on, and you feel like seeing him it's fine to say 'Yes' to last-minute plans. If you are worried that he is taking you for granted, address it directly: 'I enjoy seeing you, but when you ask me out at the last minute I feel like an afterthought. Could you give me more notice next time?'

DOING SINGLE WELL: YOUR DYSFUNCTIONAL DATING RULES

Whether we have read dating rulebooks or not, we all develop our own subconscious rulebook. Some of it we pick up from our families, some from the media, some from friends. Not all our rules are dysfunctional. For example, "be kind" is generally a good one (unless your date is very rude and unkind)! But there are a lot of rules that we could definitely do without.

In order to identify the rules that might be operating for you and stopping you from being your most authentic self while dating, think about your "shoulds." To identify them, it might help to think about the things you would hate to do, or that would make you feel guilty or embarrassed on a date. Alternatively, think about the things you've criticized yourself for when past dates haven't worked out.

Some dysfunctional dating rules I've had or heard:

- I should offer to split the bill and protest if he insists on paying – allowing him to pay means I am beholden to him.

- I should not wear wedges and should always wear a skirt – men don't like wedges and they like legs.

- I should never cancel – I should go even if I don't feel like it.

- I should always show interest in what he has to say.

- I should accept his touch, and kiss him if he wants to kiss me, even if I don't feel like it – it's only a kiss.

- I shouldn't monopolize the conversation – I should ask about him.

- I shouldn't seem too keen – it makes me seem desperate.

- I shouldn't have sex with him on the first date – he'll think I'm a slut.

- I should have sex with him after three dates – he'll think I'm frigid if I don't.

Post your own "shoulds" on Facebook @doingsinglewell

THE AMBIGUITY OF DATING

As we discussed before, part of the reason why rulebooks are so compelling is they promise to reduce the ambiguity that is a part of all dating experiences. Few people like ambiguity and uncertainty when it comes to situations where they are vulnerable and putting themselves on the line. If you are someone who related to being an island or a wave in the previous chapter, then the world of dating can be extra tricky – like visiting another country and not knowing the language. Have you caught yourself thinking any of these?

'Why didn't he call?'

'Is he dating other people?'

'Does he really like me?'

'Is he "the one"?'

We have all had, or heard someone express, these anxieties. In the most distressed of single women, thoughts like these can become obsessive and interrupt their ability to concentrate on other things. Rather than living their own wonderful lives, these ladies spend countless hours doing things aimed at reducing their anxiety. Things like: stalking their dates online, compulsively checking their phones, emails, social media and dating accounts, and asking friends, *'What do you think he means by this text?!'* can feel like a good idea at the time but usually just keep us stuck in an anxiety rut.

Unfortunately, in this technological dating age, ambiguity is becoming even more pronounced. Communicating in written form via text message or email reduces the amount of cues we can use to glean an accurate interpretation of our date's true feelings or intent. The advent of internet dating has increased everyone's access to new dating prospects and (for both good and bad) made dating multiple people easier. Even the sorts of relationships we form can be more varied. Social media such as Facebook and Instagram also give us access to ambiguous information about our dates, that we would otherwise have been protected from until we developed more security and trust in the relationship.

Modern dating technologies also allow for "minimal-effort" dating. Because texts and emails are so easily sent, little effort needs to go into them, and therefore the meaning of that effort can be ambiguous. Men and women who are ambivalent about dating someone can string the relationship along, "breadcrumbing" their dates, as it requires relatively little time. Similarly, compared to the discomfort of ending the dating relationship, many people prefer the minimal effort of "ghosting" over clean and unambiguous endings and closures.

So how do we navigate such a dating landscape and remain sane?

1. Notice worst-case thinking and learn to generate alternatives

Every time you catch yourself feeling bad about a dating scenario, ask yourself:

'Do I really know that my interpretation of this situation is right?'

'Do I have any evidence against this interpretation of the events?'

'What are three other explanations that could explain this event?'

2. Minimize ambiguity

– Call or meet up in person rather than text or email.

– Ask to meet an internet date sooner rather than later.

– Make what you are looking for in a relationship clear, both on your internet profile and in what you say about yourself on dates Remember, if you do want a serious relationship, hiding the truth and trying to play it cool is a bad strategy. It will only scare off men who want what you really want, and keep the unsuitable ones interested.

– And social media. *Do not* add your date as a friend on your socials until you have a very well-established relationship. Wait until you've formed the sort of bond where you feel comfortable asking him about anything on his social pages that you are unsure or uncomfortable about. Similarly, if things don't work out, agree to delete each other off social media. This can be a temporary measure if desired, but it is important to minimize any temptation to check.

3. Minimize checking and reassurance seeking

– Set strict rules for yourself around when to check your phone and email

e.g. *I'll only check my phone / email if I hear a message come in.*

or *I'll check my phone / email twice a day at 12pm and 5pm.*

– Notice and resist the urge to stalk him on the internet. Many of the below questions may help talk you out of it:

'Do I really want to be learning about him this way? What if I learn something bad and then feel stuck asking about it because he'll know I was checking up on him?'

'Is this how I want to spend my time? If he asked me what I did today, would I want to say "stalk you"... or something else?'

'What happened last time I did this? Did it really make me feel better / more secure in the relationship?'

'From my own experience, is what is on the internet about me a *true* representation of what is going on in my world?' (Often, we are very selective about what is in the public realm and therefore any information gleaned is likely to be skewed or inaccurate.)

–Do not ask the people around you to interpret anything for you. They know even less about the guy than you do!

Yes, you might respect their advice, but their advice can only be based on their experiences and ideas. And those experiences will be different. (A bit like comparing Romeo and Juliet's situation with Brad and Angelina's!) In fact, any similarities you might find are likely to be purely coincidence!

You will find that everyone will have good intentions when trying to offer advice. However, the information you gain from various sources will likely contradict itself and just leave you confused.

4. Communicate!

Part of forming a healthy relationship is learning how to talk with each other about your needs and feelings. If you have doubts or questions, try to be brave and speak about them as soon as possible. Doing so in a vulnerable, non-accusatory way will not scare off the right sort of partner. Make sure you use "I" language, rather than "you" language and be *specific*.

E.g. *'I feel disappointed when you say you want to meet up with me on the weekend and then I don't hear from you until Sunday night,'* rather than: *'You never follow through!'*

5. If all else fails use this guideline: If it is not a clear 'Yes' then the answer is 'No.'

The above statement is not always true. However, some people find that it is preferable to have closure around a relationship rather than being kept in limbo about it. It might be that if trying the above strategies doesn't work to calm your anxiety, then the relationship causing the anxiety isn't the relationship for you. Perhaps, given your own relationship history or attachment patterns, this guy is just not capable of giving you the consistent feedback and attention you need. If you have tried talking about what you need to no avail, and you feel like he continues to give you mixed messages, ending the relationship may be the more self-caring option.

Many single women will tell me that when they met the right person for them, dating became easy. They were no longer in any doubt of their date's feelings for them, and felt confident to ask for what they needed. As such, there was far less stress and anxiety and things just seemed to flow. If things aren't flowing for you, and you have tried to manage your anxiety, then perhaps the problem isn't you. If it's not a clear 'Yes' from him, then it might be best Cassuming it's a 'No' and ending it.

CHAPTER 16

THE BAD DATING FEELINGS

The main reason we aren't as authentic as we would like to be is that we can experience some pretty yucky emotions when we try to behave in an authentic way if that means going against our personal rulebook. These emotions are generally guilt, embarrassment (or fear of embarrassing ourselves), and social anxiety.

GUILT

'I don't want to have sex, but I shouldn't stop now, that would just be a tease.'

Guilt is the feeling we get when we believe – accurately or not – that we have done something, or that we're about to do something, that might cause harm to another person. It's our conscience which measures our behavior against the rulebook in our head.

Guilt can help us maintain our relationships but only when the signals it sends are accurate. The difficulty is that sometimes our rulebooks are unnecessarily strict or focused on what is good for others, rather than what is good for us. Having a lot of guilt can indicate that we have too high standards for ourselves, or prioritize others' needs over our own. Research has found that, possibly due to socialization, women seem to suffer more from this habitual form of guilt. And, like an overly sensitive smoke detector, when our trigger for guilty feelings is set too low, our guilt alarm can go off just as much when we do the dating equivalent of burning the toast, as when the whole relationship house is on fire!

Over time, too much guilt can erode our self-esteem, making us overly apologetic and leaving us feeling unentitled to voice any complaints, or unable to set healthy boundaries. We can also develop the tendency to prioritize other people's happiness and satisfaction over our own. As such, when feeling guilty, single women can tend to suppress their own wants and do things out of obligation rather than because they really want to. This reduces authenticity but also makes dating (and life) much less enjoyable and more hard work than it needs to be.

Sometimes it's hard to determine whether our guilt is valid and should be listened to, or if it's habitual, as a result of high standards or self-sacrifice. Next time you feel guilty try the following:

1. Identify the "should" or personal rule that you have violated to cause the guilt.

2. Ask yourself the following questions:

- Does this rule apply *all* the time?

- Is this rule in my best interests at this time?

- If the situation were reversed what would I want the other person to do?

3. Identify what you would like to do if you were being really honest, and ask yourself: How would I express this without being a bitch?

Have a look at the following examples and then have a go yourself! Post your examples on our Facebook page @doingsinglewell

Anna

1. The rule I have is: 'I should give everyone a chance if they show interest in me.'

2. This rule doesn't apply *all* the time. For example, I'd never consider going out with a married man even if he was interested in me. It's also not in my best interests to go out with this guy as I'd just be wasting an evening that I could be spending doing something I enjoy or even meeting someone who I do connect with more. I'd never want a guy to go out with me out of pity if the situation were reversed!

3. If I were being honest I'd like to tell him I'm not interested in going out with him as I've found his text messages inconsistent and dismissive.

Grace

1. The rule I have is: 'I should treat everyone with respect.'

2. This rule applies most of the time, except maybe where I'm not being treated with respect. This rule (with that exception) is in my best interests as I want to feel good about myself and be known as someone with integrity. I would like someone to treat me with respect if the situation were reversed.

3. If I were being honest, I would call him and apologize for getting drunk and disappearing on him, leaving him with the bill. I would tell him that I'm not proud of my behavior and that he deserved better. I would also have to say though that I don't think I'm in the right place, emotionally, to be dating, and that I don't think we should see each other again.

If you feel like you need more help with this I highly recommend: *The Life-Changing Magic of not Giving a F**k* (2016) by Sarah Knight.

EMBARRASSMENT

'OMG I can't believe I had parsley stuck in my teeth that whole date!'

Embarrassment is a temporary emotion that tells us that we accidentally failed to behave according to perceived social standards. Embarrassment is usually short-lived and eventually funny – unless the "not good enough" gremlins get hold of it and use it to tell us that we are pathetic! Embarrassment is always linked to wanting to be liked, and the fear that others might judge us negatively for a mistake.

Faux pas, social gaffes, blunders, putting our foot-in-our-mouth, being gauche, and bungling – if the quantity of terms we have to describe social errors indicates anything, it indicates how commonplace it is to make them. According to researchers, the most common experiences that trigger embarrassment are: tripping and falling, spilling drinks and food, ripping pants or having wardrobe malfunctions, accidental flatulence or belching, forgetting the names of others, and having your private thoughts or feelings exposed and receiving undesired attention. Given that list, is it any wonder that embarrassment is so common among daters? The social world is complex, and there as many unwritten social rules as there are social situations. Part of being authentic is to accept that we are all imperfect and are going to make mistakes, and as such, to be kind to ourselves when this inevitably happens.

The trick with embarrassment is to firstly realize that you and what you do are not as important or memorable as you may think! The "spotlight effect" is the name given to the fact that people overestimate the extent to which their appearance and actions are noticed and remembered by others. We tend to stew on embarrassing situations, playing them over and over in our heads, but the reality is that the other people who witnessed it will have likely forgotten it already!

Being authentic means trying to embrace the situation and find the humor in it. Practicing telling our tales of embarrassment in the spirit of entertaining others can help us open up to the idea that we are likeable even when we aren't perfect and even because of our funny mistakes! When we don't take ourselves so seriously and can laugh at the stupid things that can happen, the "not good enough" gremlins can't use these things against us to turn embarrassment into shame. And, when we are open to being embarrassed, we can give ourselves permission to be our true selves, and not put on a show, or play a role while dating.

DOING SINGLE WELL: BEST WORST-DATE STORY

Have a think about the best worst-dating experience you've had where you or something you did was at least partially to blame. It's easy to tell tales where other people play the comic role, but much harder and more vulnerable to share something that paints you as the goofball. Write it out in a humorous way and post it on our Facebook page @doingsinglewell

'I decided to go home with this guy I'd been dating. He was super-hot and funny, and I felt we had a good connection ... We were getting busy on his perfect white bed. I was so into him I didn't stop to think about how erm, "moist" everything was. It was only when it was all over that I looked down and got the biggest shock! I had gotten my period and there was mess everywhere! Buckets of it! I was so mortified I actually ran into the bathroom and locked myself in ... He was very nice about it though, and

we were able to laugh about it after a shower, and me offering to buy him new sheets!' – Casey, 27 years old.

SOCIAL ANXIETY

'What if I say something stupid?'

A certain amount of social anxiety is a normal part of dating. We all worry about what others think, and we want to be liked. Who doesn't want the guy they have the hots for to return the sentiment?! It is actually a sign that things are going well, and you are suitably interested in him! Being anxious means that you care! The problem occurs when we don't know how to calm ourselves down, so we experience dating as extremely unpleasant, avoid it altogether, or can't be ourselves because of the level of nervous tension.

Single women with a lot of "not good enough" gremlins will be more prone to social anxiety. It makes sense – if we have a lot of shame and feel there is something wrong with us, of course we are going to be more anxious about how people view us. Because single women with social anxiety worry about saying and doing the wrong thing, they can be prone to over-thinking and rehearsing so that they come across as disingenuous – it's hard to have an authentic reaction to something our date has said when we are too preoccupied thinking about what we should say next! Avoiding eye contact for fear of being exposed, going blank and not knowing what to say, or making minimal, trite, or inexpressive responses for fear of saying something stupid can give our date the impression that we are aloof and disinterested. On the opposite, but no more authentic, end of the spectrum, a lot of people with social anxiety rely on alcohol to help them loosen up. Though a glass of wine may be fine, alcohol is not necessarily the greatest good-decision serum in larger quantities!

So, instead of booze and bad jokes, when dating with social anxiety try to:

1. Find a strategy to help you calm down before a date. You might download a meditation app, do some slow breathing or muscle relaxation, anything that lowers your heart rate and interrupts your panicky thoughts about the date.

2. Remind yourself that anxiety is normal and he's probably feeling it too!

3. Remind yourself that you are looking for someone who likes you for you, and that this is possible! Your family likes you (most of the time) and your friends do too, so why wouldn't he?!

4. Own your anxiety if you need to! Studies have found that naming emotions can help regulate them, so saying 'Geez, I'm really nervous tonight!' can break the ice with him and also help you stay calm.

5. Practice: The good thing about dating apps is there are plenty of people out there you can practice dating on. Try not to put too much pressure on any one date and use dates as practice sessions until you start to feel more comfortable.

... And remember, if social anxiety is affecting your life in a very big way, then do invest in yourself and get help. There are very good psychological treatments for social anxiety; it is not something you have to just suffer through.

DOING SINGLE WELL: THE AUTHENTICITY CHOICE POINT

Think of a recent experience on a date, or with a friend, family member, or work colleague where you weren't authentic, or didn't say or do something you wanted to. Run the movie of this interaction in your head and pause at the point of choice: where you could have chosen to be authentic but didn't. Ask yourself the following questions and have a look at Jennie's example:

Jennie picked the time that she was on a date with a guy she liked, but he had chosen a really noisy restaurant ... She had suffered through the date but wasn't really "there" in the way she wanted to be, as she was getting more and more frustrated with the sound levels. She paused the movie at the point at which they had been seated, given menus, and ordered a glass of wine.

1. What am I afraid will happen if I am truthful and share my experience, or do what I want to do with this person?

I am afraid I might offend him. He has gone to a lot of trouble to pick and book this restaurant and I should appreciate it.

2. How will I feel if I don't share what I'm thinking and feeling, or stop myself from doing what I want to do?

I will feel agitated and begin to tune out. I will get resentful and want to cut the night short.

3. If I weren't feeling anxious, guilty, or embarrassed what would I most want to say to this person? What would I most want to do?

If I didn't feel guilty I would tell him I want to leave.

4. How could I make this vulnerability both kind to myself and to the other person?

I would tell him that I really enjoy his company and appreciate the effort he went to in booking the restaurant, but that I want to go somewhere quieter, so we can really have the chance to connect.

CHAPTER 17

DATING WITH AUTHENTICITY

Whether you have decided to stay single, or are interested in dating, living an authentic life is paramount to Doing Single Well. Trimberger (2005) suggests that developing "autonomy" is a key component to long-term life satisfaction for single and for coupled women. I propose that the three-step journey of knowing ourselves, compassionately owning our "stuff," and setting boundaries results in the kind of freedom, self-determination, and self-fulfillment that is at the heart of autonomy. However, I prefer to use the terminology "authenticity" because I think it captures the very important aspects of self-love and self-acceptance which are not inherent in autonomy. As flagged in Chapter 15, the journey to authenticity, as I see it, has three parts:

1. Knowing yourself

A lot of the information within these pages has provided us with ways to get to know ourselves and the "stuff" we get stuck in. It is important that we know our stuff as, like a dirty window pane, it is impossible to see our reflection clearly when we are all grimy with stuff. We also can't see how awesome, brilliant, and technicolor life beyond the dirt is!

When we carry around man myths, while also yearning for a relationship, we catch ourselves in a double-bind. It's hard feeling resentful, hopeless, and cynical, and especially so when we position the cause of those feelings outside of our control – we can't change "men!" Ungluing ourselves means dropping our man myths and seeing men as people, with all the same hopes, fears, and insecurities that we have. Even if we don't want a relationship, this will still be helpful – men are 50% of the population so we are bound to run into a few!

Similarly, when our heads are riddled with gremlins, we will fall over ourselves when it comes to living happily single or having a great time dating. How can we have a great time doing anything with the voices in our head telling us that we have had our chance, we are too picky, our time is running out, we stuffed up or we are unworthy?! It is essential that we get to know our gremlins and learn how to befriend them so that they lose their bite.

Once we are free of man myths and gremlins, we can start to see ourselves for the wonderful women that we are. Only then can we view our situation as a single woman clearly. We can assess whether we really do want a relationship, or whether we are avoiding, and we can begin the task of living (and dating) with love and integrity. When we aren't stuck in shame and "not good enough" beliefs we can truly enjoy who we are, in all our beautiful, imperfect complexity. Because we feel worthy, we can prioritize putting the effort into ourselves: building our tribe, caring for ourselves, finding our purpose, and meeting our own needs as a priority. When we meet all our own emotional and physical needs, we are no longer depriving or abandoning ourselves, and we can feel truly satisfied with life in a way that has nothing to do with being in a relationship or not. We become our own life partner and best friend.

Without any of that stuff in the way, our own positive personalities can shine through, and we are able to more rationally see our dates for who they are. What is more, when we understand our stuff on a relational level: our family programs of what love is, the chemistry of love, our chemical signatures, and our attachment patterns, we are more likely to make healthy choices for ourselves, rather than feel lost in a never-ending cycle of bad relationships.

2. Owning your stuff

Remember that hiding our "stuff" by "faking it," or following rules will never serve us well. Who wants to end up committed to a guy who isn't suited to us?! We need to be ourselves while dating so that the guy who will love that person wholeheartedly gets a chance to meet and choose her!

We all want to be liked, and it's tempting to try to change ourselves, or pretend to be someone we're not, to gain love or approval. But if we just mirror everything a guy says he wants, and bend ourselves pretzel-like to fit in with him, we are far more likely to fall into either of two traps:

Firstly, we might turn a relationship-ready guy off – it's a bit boring dating a mirror! Having some areas where we are different will generally be more interesting to him. We will have better conversation, and we'll be more memorable. Most people are looking for partnerships that bring out the best in themselves, and give opportunities to grow. One of the joys of dating is becoming more than we are by ourselves. This is only possible when we date someone who is brave enough to be an individual, and will contribute an authentic perspective in a relationship!

The second trap we can fall into when not being authentic is attracting someone who is self-absorbed, or a relationship perfectionist, who consequently isn't relationship-ready. If someone is pleased by how accommodating we are (without trying to accommodate us equally), and / or puts us on a pedestal because he thinks we are "perfect,", we might indeed be dating someone who won't be able to handle the relationship when the honeymoon period is over, and the inevitable differences emerge.

Working so hard at being likeable, being attractive in a superficial way, and playing by the rules can be exhausting. When we forego trying to please our date quite so much, we gain energy and self-assurance. We can get pleasure in dating, as in life.

Just because you know your stuff doesn't mean it will magically disappear. Some of it has been around since your childhood, and like a stubborn mark, no amount of scrubbing can rid you of it totally. And that's fine! Great, even!

Who are we without our foibles and neuroses? Is there anyone you can name who is a perfect person?

Just as life has marked your body with freckles, scars, grey hair, stretch marks, and wrinkles, your experiences have made you the person you are today. Accepting this, and even embracing it, is the key to undermining the power it has over you. When you know and own your stuff, you learn to respond to it, rather than to react to it in an automatic, knee-jerk kind of way. Take the below examples:

Jane was at dinner with her date. Things were going well until the waiter asked them if they'd like dessert. They both took a menu and kept chatting. When the waiter came around again, Jane ordered the chocolate mousse. Her date said he would pass on dessert. Jane immediately felt heat rush to her face and a sick feeling in the pit of her stomach. Her head was telling her she was greedy and indulgent, and that "no one would want to be with a fat girl"... She paused, took a deep breath, and let out a nervous laugh. 'I'm sorry,' she said. 'I just had a moment... when you didn't order dessert I had a flashback to my horrible sister telling me I was a greedy-guts. I need to let you know because otherwise I won't be able to enjoy the chocolate!'

Her date laughed, and told her about how refreshing he found it that she ate. He said he'd been on many dates with women who picked at their food and he found it both strange and embarrassing when the waiter would ask if there was anything wrong! Jane immediately relaxed and felt the tension drain out of her. Her chest felt warm and open, and she felt closer to her date than she could have imagined before. Even if he didn't call her again, she knew it wouldn't be because of her weight. That was just her old "not good enough" gremlin. She was pleased she had been brave and raised it, because she knew it would have ruined her night, made her more preoccupied, could have shut her down at the time, and caused her to worry incessantly afterwards.

*

Kasey knew it as soon as the guy she had been seeing "passed the test" ... it was this thing with her where the moment she became seriously interested in a guy she became a monster! Finding herself stalking his Instagram feed, purely because he hadn't immediately responded to her text was all the information she needed to know he was now "the one" (at least her crazy attachment brain thought so!). She also knew she was in for a rough ride.

With a small smile she stood up and marched out of her office. She told her secretary that she didn't want to be disturbed for the rest of the afternoon and asked her to mind her phone. She then went back to work and every time she had thoughts about him, and what he was doing, she rolled her eyes at them and then regained her focus.

When she did speak with him later that night, she told him that because of some experiences she'd had in the past she was sensitive to rejection. She said that she felt insecure when her texts went unanswered and, because she didn't want him to have to change his patterns, just because of her "stuff," she suggested that she was going to refrain from texting during the day and instead call him after work. She could tell he was a little confused, but he readily agreed that after-work chats worked better for him too. They spent the next hour chatting, and by the time she hung up she had a nice feeling in her heart, and was looking forward to seeing him the following Friday night.

*

Anne wasn't a ditherer, but she sure was dithering! She had tried on five different outfits and asked her teenage daughter which one made her look younger. 'At least she hadn't gone ahead and booked that Botox appointment,' she thought, with a shake of her head! Her ex-husband had been a dick when he had run off with his much younger secretary, but she wasn't going to stick needles in her face because of him! When she went into the bathroom she took a good look at herself – the laughter lines around her eyes and the dark spots on her face which had never really evened out after her last pregnancy. This was her face. It showed her life, and she was not going to be ashamed of it. She put on minimal makeup – she hardly wore it anyway, put on her comfortable-but-nice shoes and headed out the door before she could lose her nerve!

He was waiting for her at the restaurant and stood up for her as she arrived. 'Phew,' she caught herself thinking. 'At least I must look like my photo!' She smiled again at the pesky thought ... it had snuck up out of nowhere! They sat, and the conversation flowed easily. He was both considerate and charming. He had a quirky sense of humor too, just the type she liked. Things were going so well that she couldn't quite work out why, over the next hour, the anxiety within her grew. It wasn't until the very pretty young waitress with the low-cut shirt asked him if he would like to see the wine menu again that she had the light bulb moment. She was feeling insecure ... she was feeling like he was too good for her! She was wondering why he would be interested in an "old chook" like her!

The date drew to a close, and as they were waiting for her taxi, she took both of his hands and turned to him. 'I had a really nice time tonight and would like to see you again,' she said sincerely, looking into his eyes. He squeezed her hands and let out a breath she hadn't been aware he was holding. 'I'm so glad to hear you say that! It's not often I get to meet someone I connect with so well.' She smiled and said 'I'm glad to hear you say that … I was worried you wouldn't be interested when you saw how old I was!' He looked surprised and said, 'I'm too old to be bothered about age!'

*

Okay, be honest, did reading those make you cringe at times? Being truly honest is *hard*! It's vulnerable! But it's also the lightning-path to intimacy. We don't have to lay it all out on the first date. But knowing our stuff, keeping awareness of it while we are dating (and living), responding to it rather than reacting after it, and owning and introducing it into the dialogue with our date when necessary, is the only way we will be able to grow. Once we can own our stuff and talk about it freely, it no longer rules us. Then, we can work together with our dates against it.

I'm not saying that we need to own our stuff at the outset, nor am I saying we have to give our dates reasons for the boundaries that we set. Our timing is ours and I suggest that it should be dictated by how much our stuff is interfering in feeling happy and relaxed with our dates. For example, Kasey may have had to own her stuff early to manage her anxiety, whereas Anne may have been able to leave her disclosure until a later date without too much going badly. Generally owning our stuff will be part of the dance of gradually developing intimacy. The more both you and your date slowly reveal about yourselves and the more support and acceptance you receive from each other, the closer you will grow.

I'm also not saying that owning our stuff will always go as smoothly as it has done in my examples. There are people out there who don't like true intimacy, who will be judgmental and who will choose to see our flaws as a weakness. They might even try to use information we have given them against us to feel powerful themselves. The great news is that by owning our stuff we get to see our dates for who they are early, so that we don't waste time with them! We are who we are. They will find out all our secrets eventually, so isn't it better to be brave and vulnerable (even if it means potentially being rejected early on)? It's much easier to walk away from someone who can't respect us early on than it is after we have formed an attachment.

And P.S. *Everyone* has stuff. So yes, we can feel sorry for the guy who rejects us, or criticizes us for our vulnerability. He's going to have a very lonely life in the search of the "perfect" partner!

The trick with owning our stuff is to give enough information in an unambiguous way to help our date understand where we are coming from, and what we need. Owning our stuff generally involves these parts:

1. Trigger: Speak about this factually without emotion-laden language, e.g. 'When I'm waiting alone for you ...' *not* 'When I'm sitting here like a mug for ages ...!'

2. Feeling: Use the "I" pronoun not "you" e.g. 'I feel anxious' *not* 'You give me anxiety.'

3. Belief (or stuff that has been triggered): Show insight that you know these are thoughts, not real facts e.g. 'These silly thoughts keep coming up for me that I couldn't possibly be young enough for you,' not 'I'm not young enough for you!'

4. History related to that stuff: You don't have to be detailed, and you can add this into later conversations if you wish. Just keep in mind that you are looking for him to understand where you are coming from, so the more information the better.

5. What you need: Request, don't demand: 'I'd like it if you could text me if you are running late,' *not* 'You need to send a text next time!'

We don't have to deal with all five aspects of owning our stuff all at once in the same breath, or even the same conversation. That would be the equivalent to floodlighting our stuff when all we really need is to hold a little candle up to illuminate some parts of it. However, if the relationship continues, we will need to address them all at some stage so we can ensure we are on the same page as our date. Because our stuff is fairly enduring it's good to get well practiced with each of these five aspects so that you understand how best to talk about them, if and when the need arises. Using the examples above:

JANE	1. Trigger: When I ordered dessert and you didn't.
	2. Feeling: I felt shame and anxiety.
	3. Belief: I had thoughts like 'I'm greedy, fat, and unattractive.'
	4. History: Just like when my sister used to tease me about being fat.
	5. What she needs: I'd love it if you could share my dessert to make me feel better.
KASEY	1. Trigger: When I didn't get a reply to my text.
	2. Feeling: I felt anxious and insecure.
	3. Belief: Although I know it was in my head, I worried that you had gone cold on us and had decided you weren't interested in seeing me again.
	4. History: My dad was a drinker and I never knew where I stood with him. One minute I was a golden child, the next minute he would be giving me the silent treatment.
	5. What she needs: I'd feel better if there was less uncertainty in our communication. I wonder if we could just plan to call each other after work so then I know what to expect?
ANNE	1. Trigger: When I started dating again.
	2. Feeling: I felt shame and anxiety.
	3. Belief: I couldn't help but think: 'Men want younger women,' and 'I'm not young or attractive enough.'
	4. History: Because my ex-husband left me for a much younger woman.
	5. What she needs: I need a man who I can rely on, and who I know loves me for who I am, inside and out.

WHOSE STUFF? YOUR STUFF!

Please note that although it is nice if your partner can help you meet your needs, never forget that it is not his responsibility to do so. When we date a new person, we inherit their baggage and they inherit ours. That is the unglamorous fact that famous couples therapist Dan Wile talked about when he said (and I paraphrase) when you choose a partner, you are choosing a bag of unsolvable problems, the key to a successful relationship is choosing problems that you can live with the rest of your life!

So please don't get lazy and start blaming him for your feelings. Your feelings are yours, they come from your body, and are more often than not, largely due more to your history than anything happening in the present time with you and your date. Owning your stuff means owning this fact and not projecting the responsibility or blame for your feelings onto your partner.

For example:

Kasey had had a stressful week. When she got to the wine bar, she ordered a much-needed glass of Riesling. Ten minutes later she began to get agitated … Where was he? Fifteen minutes and a full glass of wine later, she was just about to get her bag and storm out when he came in looking harried. 'Where were you?!' she demanded. 'I've been waiting here for ages!' He looked taken aback and his shoulders squared. 'It's only a few minutes!' he defended.

Compared with:

Kasey had had a stressful week. When she got to the wine bar, she ordered a much-needed glass of Riesling. Ten minutes later she began to get agitated … Where was he? Fifteen minutes and a full glass of wine later she noticed her anger and the urge to throw a tantrum. She closed her eyes and took some deep breaths. She reminded herself how busy they both were at work and how difficult it was to get anywhere at rush hour... It wasn't that he didn't care. When he tapped her on the shoulder, she opened her eyes with an ironic smile. She gave him a kiss on the cheek and said, 'I'm sorry in advance if I seem a bit antsy, I know you must have been held up, but your being late triggered my abandonment stuff and I was working myself up into a right lather!' He smiled and gave her a giant hug. 'It's good to see you,' he said. She smiled too. 'Yes, I've missed you!'

What you will notice is that whenever your stuff sneaks under your radar and leaks out, and it will, you will be imperfect – it will come out as one of the Gottman's "Four horsemen of the apocalypse." The four horsemen refer to the unhelpful communication patterns that were shown in research to predict the end of the relationship. They are:

Criticism: An attack on your partner's character, not just their behavior, usually packaged as "You always …" or "You never …" statements. The implication is that your partner is offensive, not just that he has offended you.

"You men are all the same, superficial, cradle-snatching, skirt-chasers … I saw the way you were flirting with that waitress!"

Defensiveness: Occurs usually in response to a perceived attack or criticism. It usually takes the form of righteous indignation, innocent victimhood, counter-attack, and whining. It has the effect of pushing the blame back on to your partner: 'The problem isn't me, it's you.'

'I don't always order dessert. You should have told me you weren't going to!'

Contempt: A statement that conveys a lack of respect and a superiority over your partner. It can include mocking, sarcasm, eye rolling, and mimicking.

'Trust you to be late! Don't know how to tell the time yet, heh?' (Mimicking) 'I'm Eddie and I'm too busy and important to worry about the time!'

Stonewalling: When one partner withdraws from the interaction and shuts down. This is not necessarily done to punish your partner, but just because you feel overwhelmed, ashamed, criticized, or worried that if you said anything, you'd make it worse.

Jane's date: 'Is there something wrong? You've hardly touched your dessert.'

Jane: 'No …' (Her eyes remain downcast and she keeps playing with her food.)

If you want to know more about these patterns and how to overcome them, have a look online, or read any number of the

Gottman books – Seven Principles *For Making a Marriage Work* (1999) is still one of my favorites.

3. Setting boundaries

Setting boundaries is the final stage of dating with authenticity. A boundary is declaring what is okay and what is not okay. Brené Brown says having clear boundaries is the key to self-love and being able to treat others with loving kindness. If we don't set boundaries, we end up resenting others, and switching off to our partner, and to life more generally.

In our culture, we are not comfortable setting boundaries. We are taught to please and be agreeable. We want everyone to like us, and we don't want to disappoint people. Even as kids, we are told to eat things we don't like, to hug relatives even if we don't want to, and even sometimes, to play sports and study subjects at school because our parents think that they are important.

As a grown-up, once we know our stuff and have owned our stuff, we then have the right, the insight, and the freedom to set our own boundaries. Keep in mind that everyone has different comfort zones in different areas because we all have different stuff. Just because you need to set a boundary around something that you haven't heard anyone else have a boundary for, that doesn't make it wrong or unnecessary. Similarly, just because your date has never had to do things in quite that way before, doesn't mean it is unreasonable to ask.

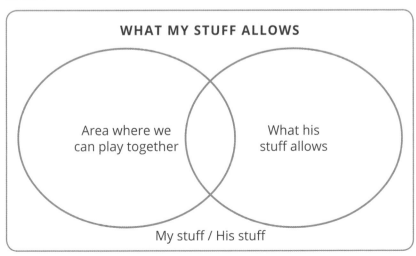

Whether our date will be able to willingly meet our needs and abide by our boundary really depends on the intersection between our stuff and his stuff. For example, you might have stuff around feeling unimportant or ignored, and feel triggered if he continues to check his phone while you are together. He might have stuff about not being available for his kids due to feelings of shame about his divorce and separation from them. Given the conflicting needs of your stuff and his stuff it might be that it does not work out between you two.

I don't like the word "compromise" when it comes to our boundaries. Often when we try to compromise we step out of "willingness." Willingness is a genuine, clearly-felt openness to do something. It is *not* saying 'Yes' to make him feel guilty, to please him, because we feel we should compromise, or to avoid conflict. Any compromise we make needs to feel as good as our original preference.

A silly example: If I went to buy ice cream and ordered a dark chocolate sorbet, and the ice-cream man said, 'Sorry, we don't have that today, but I can give you dark-mint-chocolate,' that would be fine! I'd be totally willing to do that, as to me, dark-choc-mint is just as good as dark chocolate. If he'd said strawberry, or butterscotch, or rocky-road, or even milk chocolate, I wouldn't be so willing – it just wouldn't feel the same. I'd prefer to go without. It would be a compromise that crosses my felt preference or my boundaries. If I were doing the Boundary Bagel exercise in Chapter 5, "dark chocolate" would be in my inflexible area and 'other flavors in addition to dark chocolate' would be in my flexible area. Considering what we can happily accept and what makes us feel uncomfortable, "switched off," disappointed, resentful, or stressed can help us work out where our boundaries are.

In the above dating example, you may not be able to willingly accept his ongoing divided attention. It might not be respectful of yourself, or authentic to your needs and feelings. Perhaps "Undivided attention at the dinner table" would be in the inflexible area of your Boundary Bagel. Also, he may not be able to willingly make himself unavailable for his kids – it might take him out of self-respect, and it might compromise his authentic needs and feelings.

"Having his phone switched on in case of emergency" might be in his inflexible area of his Boundary Bagel. Of course, raising this issue and talking about your flexible and inflexible areas respectfully might mean you are more likely to find an area of overlap with him – something that you can both agree to willingly. However, this turf needs to be navigated very carefully so that we don't trick ourselves into crossing our own boundaries out of an effort to collaborate with our dates. If we cross our own boundary we'll end up feeling resentful over time, and it might come out in passive aggressive behavior, sniping at him, feeling turned off him, numbness, or even depression.

Boundaries can change over time, especially with developing trust and security in a relationship. In fact, a secure relationship with a partner who compassionately helps us move through our stuff by helping "right the wrongs" that caused it, is one of the most effective ways to heal. Unfortunately, one of the most effective ways to stay stuck in our stuff is to repeat it again and again by not saying 'No' and not setting boundaries.

In the above example, you would get angrier and more resentful if he continued to prioritize checking his phone and his kids. Your sense that you are unlovable and unworthy of being someone's top priority would grow, and eventually, you may even act out in a childish or petulant way and elicit scolding, criticism, or contempt which would further reinforce your lack of lovability.

When we are looking for our boundaries in our dating life, we need to keep in mind that boundaries apply in many areas:

- **Material boundaries:** Our comfort level and rules around giving, lending, borrowing, or taking things (e.g. money, clothes, food, books, car, toothbrush).

- **Physical boundaries:** Our body, five senses, personal space, and privacy rules. Who we feel comfortable kissing, hugging, and shaking hands with. How we feel about loud music, strong scents / perfumes, nudity, locked doors ... even seeing someone chew with their mouth open!

- **Sexual boundaries:** Our comfort level with sexual touch, talk, images, and activity. The who, what, where, when, and how of our sexual preferences.

- **Mental boundaries:** Our thoughts, values, and opinions. Do you know what you believe? Can you hold to your opinions, or are you easily suggestible? Can you listen with an open mind without becoming rigid? If you become argumentative, emotional, or defensive, you may have weak mental boundaries.

- **Emotional boundaries:** Our own emotions are the ones we need to take responsibility for, and we should have boundaries around taking responsibility for anyone else's emotions. Boundaries here prevent giving advice, blaming or accepting blame. If you feel guilty for someone's else's feelings, or take another's comments personally, you may have weak boundaries in this area.

- **Spiritual boundaries:** Our beliefs and experiences in connection with God or a higher power.

DOING SINGLE WELL: MARK OUT YOUR BOUNDARIES

In the above six areas make a list of your boundaries. Your boundaries separate your likes from your dislikes; the things you are and aren't willing to engage in; the things you would be willing to accept from the things that make you uncomfortable. Write them down here:

Here are some signs that your boundaries need adjusting:

- Feeling responsible for others' emotions

- Taking on the moods or emotions of others around you

- Not knowing what you really need or feel

- Worrying about what others think to the point of discounting your own thoughts, opinions, and intuition

- Worrying that if you set a boundary, it will jeopardize the relationship

- Fearing someone's anger or judgment (e.g. being called selfish or self-centered

- Finding your energy is so drained by something or someone that you neglect your own needs (including the need for food, rest, etc.)

- People-pleasing

- Avoiding intimate relationships

- Feeling unable to make decisions

- Feeling unable to say 'No'

- Feeling like you don't have rights

- Feeling anxious and guilty, or ashamed for asking for what you want

- Believing that your happiness depends on others

- Taking care of others' needs, but not your own. Or putting others' needs and feelings consistently first

- Having difficulty asking for what you want or need

- Going along with others and not doing what you want

- Being overly sensitive to criticism

- Feeling like you don't want to be a "burden"

We've discussed how to set a boundary when managing the well-meaning, and when asking for what we need. As with these boundaries, it's important to use "I statements" and begin with a request. We do not need to give reasons or explain the boundaries that we set, we have the right to say 'No' without explanation. However, in the course of a developing relationship, it can helpful to own the stuff behind our boundaries to help generate understanding and empathy.

Of course, if our boundary is not respected, it is totally appropriate to escalate to using language that is just as strong and demanding as we need. 'I'd like you to stop touching my leg' might quickly escalate to 'Get your hand off my leg!' and to standing up and walking out if needed!

With healthy boundaries, we can feel 100% in control of our circumstances. Although we can't control others, we have every confidence we can say and do the things necessary for us to have an enjoyable experience. Although setting boundaries when we are not used to doing it is not always easy – a myriad of emotions including guilt, shame and anxiety might pop up in the process – finding and setting healthy boundaries will teach us more about ourselves and help us gain more self-acceptance and self-confidence.

SEXUAL BOUNDARIES

Since the sexual revolution, women have been encouraged to enjoy their sexuality. The quirk of this is that women often now feel that they "should" be sexually active and enjoy sex.

However, women's turn-ons are often different from men's. There is a reason why pornography is largely marketed towards men, and romantic comedies towards women. Where men might get aroused by breasts, bums, lingerie, etc., women often need to feel close to their partner to feel in the mood for sex. This means that many women may not feel like becoming sexual until a fair way into a dating relationship.

Feeling like having sex is not the same as wanting to please your date, wanting to feel sexually powerful, or wanting to feel desirable. And if you don't feel like sex, that should not inspire a fear of rejection. Feeling like sex is the extension of that almost magnetic urge you have to touch the person you are flirting with. It is led by the body, not the head ... you don't think 'I want to touch their arm,' you feel the urge to do it, or, just find it happening while you are not paying attention.

So many single women I've spoken to have stepped over their own sexual boundaries. It is easy to do, because most people, both men and women, are very insecure when it comes to sex – so it is hard to say nice 'no's' without giving offence. However, as a rule of thumb, you are not ready to be sexual with a new date until you are 100% confident that, if you wanted to stop at any time, they would be respectful of this. (And respect does *not* mean sulking, keeping on trying to have sex with you, complaining, or getting angry with you. Respect means saying, 'Sure, whatever you need.') There is a great clip about consent being like a cup of tea, which I highly recommend you watch if you haven't seen it yet: https://www.youtube.com/watch?v=oQbei5JGiT8

Once you do feel drawn to have sex it is important to know how you are going to communicate your sexual needs. Dr. Rosie King talks about the "soft no sandwich" in her book *Good Loving, Great Sex* (1998). Using this method, you give a compliment or appreciate something (the top bread / softener), you say 'No' to the thing you don't like or want (the middle of the sandwich) and then you tell your partner what you'd prefer (the bottom bread / softener). For example: 'I love how passionate you are, but kissing my ears doesn't do it for me, could you kiss me here instead? Mmm, yes! Just like that!'

If you have a very sensitive and responsive partner you could soften your 'no's further by simply gently moving his kisses away from your ears and saying, 'I love it when you kiss me here.' Alternatively, if you are finding that your partner is not very responsive and your boundaries are not being respected, it is fine to escalate the strength of your 'no's: 'Stop kissing my ears.'

'I was seeing a guy for about a month when he called and told me his ex had informed him she had chlamydia, and that he should get tested. We both took the antibiotics and got told to wait for seven days before having sex again. That was fine by me, I'd never had an STD and found it a bit gross. I was totally not interested in having sex! On the other hand,

he kept texting me, telling me how horny he was. I replied saying I wasn't comfortable having sex that week, but he could come and sleep over. He said no, he was too horny, and then kept badgering me, asking me if we could use a condom, or if I could just give him oral. I put up with two days of this before I cracked it. I told him that I didn't appreciate being made to feel responsible for his sexual frustration, that I'd said 'No' and, because of his lack of respect for that, I wasn't willing to see him again.' – May, 40 years old.

CHAPTER 18

AUTHENTICITY ON THE INTERNET

Like it or not, if we want to meet a partner, it is becoming more and more likely that we'll have to experiment with using the internet. Online dating and dating apps have become commonplace and are now a normal part of many people's dating experience.

Dating authentically online can be difficult. The depersonalization of online interfaces means that it has become much easier for daters to be crass, rude, or to lie outright. And it is all too easy for some daters to lead others on, which gives online dating the bad reputation it has. However, not everyone online is a dick. Just like you may be considering online dating, so too are some good relationship-ready men, and it is silly (and limiting) to let some bad experiences sour us to what is probably the single most efficient way to meet new dates.

'I was really reluctant to try internet dating. All my friends had shared really bad stories, and I thought that it was just for hook-ups. Eventually I decided to give it a go. Henry was the first person I matched with, and the first internet date I went on. We got married 18 months later and are now expecting our first child. He is the sweetest, most reliable, and loveliest man I could imagine, the total opposite of the "players" I thought I would meet!' – Candice, 28 years old.

New online dating sites and apps are coming onto the market all the time. Their candidate pool is constantly changing, and they will often change their algorithms altering how we experience the platform. However, despite the variables, there are ways to navigate online dating to ensure we have the best experience possible:

1. Introductions only

The most important thing to remember about using any online platform is that it provides introductions only. Just like speed dating, all any online site is doing is helping us metaphorically "meet" (mostly) eligible men. This means we'll need to actually meet them in real life to determine if we have a connection. As such, I will always advise people to spend as little time as possible online with their matches. Send a few messages to determine that your match can hold a conversation, and doesn't start getting sleazy, then offer to meet them for a coffee. Don't text back and forth for weeks, as if you don't get bored, you may form false hopes and ideas about them that can leave you feeling very disappointed when you meet him in person.

'I had finally met a guy I got excited about. His messages were funny and so on-point it was almost like he knew what I was thinking. I'd gotten used to the nice habit of waking up and chatting with him before work and falling asleep wishing each other sweet dreams. I couldn't wait to meet him, but he was out of town for work and so it took a full month to line it up. You couldn't imagine my disappointment when I met him, and he looked nothing like his photos. I'm not a superficial person but he was at least 10 years older than he'd said, and had obviously poached his profile pics from the internet. That instantly broke the trust we had built, and I called it off the same day.' – Evie, 30 years old.

2. Don't judge a book by its cover

We've spoken about how choosing a partner is best based on an assessment of their character. We've also spoken about how attraction is influenced by many things, and how very little of it comes down to actual looks (the same is true for women's attraction to men as it is for men's attraction to women, as discussed in Chapter 7). Because of this, it is unwise to rule too many people out, based on their photos. Similarly, having a generous age bracket, a 5–10-year window around your current age is generally a good idea.

As a rule of thumb, say 'Yes' to anyone who looks like they would fit in with a group of your friends. For example, none of my friends have tattoos, wear leathers, or ride bikes, so it is likely I won't find much in common or develop much of an attraction to a tattooed, biker-guy. Don't say no to someone just because, based on his photo, you can't imagine kissing him, or because he is bald or short. You'll never know how you'll really feel about these things in the context of the whole person until you meet him.

'I'm a tall girl and would never normally date anyone shorter than myself. So, when I first met Chris, I was instantly turned off. I didn't want to be rude, so resigned myself to staying for dinner. Funny thing was, that by the end of the night, I'd forgotten his height. We'd had such a good time that I couldn't wait to see him again!' – Tania, 33 years old.

3. Do judge a book by its contents

Look at the photos, as well as what your potential match writes about himself for signs of what he values. Be honest with yourself – if you're not big into fitness, don't pick the guy who has three gym-selfies, no matter how hot his body is. But, once again, be generous. If you too have values of traveling or enjoying nature, you don't have to rule out a skier, just because you don't like skiing. *Who* he is will always be more important than whether or not you share the same interests.

I generally recommend making generous quick decisions, based on the "fit in with friends" criteria. Once you match, and establish that he is interested in chatting, *then* read his profile, and look at, or ask about, his values. It makes the process unnecessarily hard and discouraging to put too much work into it at the outset. Of course, this depends on your platform – if you have to pay for each message you send then you would be filtering more carefully first.

Keep in mind that educational status is unimportant if you value intellect or a good work ethic – just because he hasn't got a degree doesn't mean he isn't smart or hardworking. Career is also unimportant, excepting that it may say something about what he values. You may assume a guy who works in health values health, but my dad is a retired doctor and has been a pack-a-day smoker most of his life. So, it's best to not make snap judgments about these things! Him having kids already may actually be a great thing if you value family.

'I want a family, but I always used to say 'No' to guys who already had kids. Becoming the ugly stepmother was not an appealing prospect! Brad was honest about his two-year-old son on our first date. He talked with such love and pride about him, I was totally charmed. I could really tell that he was a family guy and a good father, not just another self-important wanker.' – Amy, 36 years old.

4. Notice sleaze and don't get sucked in

It's pretty easy to tell what a guy is looking for on the internet. He'll post half-naked photos; he may even state in his profile that he isn't looking for a relationship. Unless you are wanting a hook-up don't say 'Yes' to these guys. If it is ambiguous, you can say 'Yes' initially, then ask him when you match what he is looking for – he'll most likely tell you!

The only trap is that some guys are self-delusional – they'll say they are looking for a relationship, but their behavior will say otherwise. Suggesting coffee, not responding to late-night messages, and having a friendly (more than a flirty) tone will help you filter out the guys who only want to get off. If a guy starts messaging you in a way that is overtly sexual and you feel uncomfortable with, give him a warning: *'Hey, I'm not that sort of girl, I feel uncomfortable receiving these messages,'* and block him if he continues.

'I knew what he wanted from the moment he said, 'How about we meet at yours?' Even though he'd said on his profile he was looking for a relationship, all we ever did was have sex. It was good sex, but after a few weeks, I got bored, and wanted a more fulfilling relationship, so I ended it with him.' – Pip, 31 years old.

5. Take charge

The problem with the internet is that it takes very little effort to set up a profile. As such, many of the men you may say 'Yes' to may not actually be in the market for dating. They may have downloaded the app many months ago, and now be inactive. They may have downloaded it just for a laugh. They may even be in a relationship, and using it as fantasy material.

With free apps, it's probably safe to assume that at least 50% of the people you match with will either un-match you, or not respond to your messages. With that in mind, don't waste time. When you match with someone, begin a conversation straightaway. It doesn't have to be anything fancy, a simple, 'Hi how was your weekend?' will help you determine if the guy is actually there or not. Similarly, once you have established he is there and can hold a conversation (giving two-word answers or speaking in emojis doesn't count), ask him out. You'll find out quickly whether he makes excuses, or if he is really interested in meeting someone.

'I was getting really discouraged until I plucked up the courage to initiate the conversation. It seemed to me that no one on the app I was using actually wanted to chat to me! Once I began initiating though it got easier. There have been a lot of guys who still don't write back, but I delete them and move on, and I've have had a few good dates now.' – Tina, 39 years old.

6. Pick your platform then rotate

Different dating platforms have different advantages and disadvantages. I generally recommend single women begin by picking one that requires minimal effort and doesn't allow anyone to contact you until you've said 'Yes' to them – you don't need to be swamped by a ton of messages from inappropriate matches.

I don't think that the paid sites are any better necessarily than the free sites, so I recommend that you pick one that you like, explore it for a while, and when you find yourself getting bored or discouraged, move to another one or take a short holiday from dating. Dating requires effort, and you deserve a break every now and then.

If you are finding something discouraging while using a particular platform, then don't assume it will be the same on all platforms. Ask friends about their experiences, or try a new one to see if your issue is resolved. For example, a single woman told me about how she was having the experience that none of her matches ever responded to her messages on Bumble. She switched to Tinder and the problem was resolved. Please note, I'm not saying you should use Tinder over Bumble, this was just her experience at that time. I am suggesting that trying something new is better than stopping altogether.

You also can't underestimate the benefit of deleting your profile and starting again. Something to do with the algorithms used means that a lot of single women have been discouraged by their candidates if they've been using a platform for a long time, or have logged back on to their profile after a long break. This has been resolved when they've started afresh.

'I've been internet dating for a few years now and tried a lot of different apps. I get my favorites, but it changes. Sometimes the guys might seem more interesting on one, or I might have better conversations on another. It doesn't seem to be about whether it is paid or free or if they "match" you, or it's just based on photos. I think it's important just to stay positive and have fun with it. The minute you start complaining, you know it's time to take a break!' – Michelle, 30 years old.

7. Available men only

No guys who are overseas or still in relationships. No guys who are in your country on short-term visas or who fly-in-and-fly-out for work. I generally suggest starting with a location radius of 10km if you live in a city. If a guy is available, it will be relatively easy to line up a date. If you can't find a time within a one-week window, either one or both of you need to look at re-prioritizing your schedule! If you need a reminder of what counts as available and what doesn't, take another peek at Chapter 12.

'My relationship was going so well while my partner was at sea. He contacted me regularly and was really open about his life and his feelings. I was so excited the night before he got back for his leave I could barely sleep. The minute he landed, it felt like things were different. He cancelled plans, stopped responding to my calls and texts, and stopped sharing. For the first time since we met online he was actually here ... but he wasn't. He broke up with me three days after arriving home, and I've never seen him since. I wonder if he was actually married, and I still feel like a fool for wasting so many months on him.' – Pippa, 34 years old.

8. Be authentic!

Choose photos of the real you. To me, a nice internet dating photo is a high quality (i.e. not grainy or fuzzy) head shot of you, without sunglasses, neatly groomed, looking at the camera and smiling. I also think that adding a photo that is a full body view in normal clothes (no selfies, no bikinis, no gym) is useful.

There is nothing to be ashamed of, no matter how you think you look. There will be someone out there who finds you attractive! Choose photos that represent your values, and write about your values as well as what you're looking for in any blurb that you decide to include. If you really struggle with this, and it's stopping you from online dating, outsource the job to a close friend.

When messaging, rather than engage in inane flirtation, cut to the chase. Ask them the questions about themselves that you feel are important for you and, sooner rather than later, ask them if they are interested in meeting up for a coffee.

'I don't have a lot of photos of myself, I'm not a makeup kind of girl and never take selfies! I wasn't getting anywhere with online dating until I got my best friend to look at my profile. She took one look at my profile photo (my headshot from work) and deleted it, then uploaded some that she had of me at my birthday party. I'm okay with this, it still looks like me, and I am getting a lot more matches!' – Clarissa, 37 years old.

9. Don't take it personally

You will experience rejection, and you will reject people. This is true of all dating, but especially true of online dating. Expect it and embrace it: the people that un-match you, the messages that don't get answered, the dates that get evaded, being stood up, being ghosted, being told you aren't the one ... all of it. Just remember that every time this happens you have filtered out another poor candidate. Remember also that it is not personal. The guys that are rejecting you don't really know you at all. I like to think about being rejected in terms of it being a poor match ... it's just that sometimes my date realized it before I did.

'I used to feel awful when I was ghosted or stood up. I used to think it was because I wasn't pretty enough or interesting enough. Then I had an experience where a guy had stopped responding to me (for a week!) so I deleted the match. He tracked me down via Facebook and sent some sarcastic messages about me wasting his time and playing games. I was shocked! I found myself automatically apologizing and trying to make it better before I realized that I hadn't actually done anything wrong. From then on, I thought very differently about rejection, you just don't know what goes on in someone's head, so it's silly to even guess.' – Lilly, 29 years old.

GETTING OFFLINE AND DATING IN THE REAL WORLD

For starters, well done! Once you have actually met someone for a date you can actually begin to say you are dating! You don't know how many single women I've spoken to who have complained that they have been single for years, but when I ask them how many dates they have been on they look at me blankly. You don't get to count your single years as years of unsuccessful dating, unless you are actually ... dating!

Your mission at this stage, should you choose to accept it, is to have fun! Make dating as easy and enjoyable as possible. Suggest places that are convenient to you, and activities you'd like to do. Treat it as if you were meeting up with a good friend and put no more or less pressure on yourself than you would in that case. Treat your date no more or less well than you would a friend.

Many single women get overly freaked out about dating, putting it in the same camp as a job interview. Rather than see yourself as the interviewee, imagine you are the interviewer and you are sussing out whether you want this guy in *your* life. Use the attractiveness recipe in Chapter 7 – not to sell yourself to him, but to open him up and reveal the things you need to help you work out if he's a keeper.

- Authenticity: Be yourself.

- Attunement: Flow with him.

- Connection: "Turn towards" him and be responsive to his conversation.

Pay attention to your feelings – what is it about him that catches your curiosity? Of course, if you aren't interested in what he is saying, be authentic and kindly redirect the conversation. If you don't know about some topic, just say 'I don't know' and ask more about it. If you are tired or have had enough, tell him you are ready to leave, don't suffer through because of any "shoulds" you may have about staying a certain amount of time. Allow silences if silences occur, it's normal.

Notice any negativity you may have, thank your mind, and let it go. While you are on the date remind yourself that every experience has something positive that you can take from it. Don't allow yourself to be bored or feel discouraged, it's a sign of laziness! Be a treasure hunter and find the gems in each interaction. Sometimes it might be that you learned more about a certain topic, sometimes it might just be that you discovered a new favorite wine.

Work out beforehand what feels right for you in terms of who pays the bill, and how you want to let him know if you are keen to see him again or not. Anything goes. Pick whatever makes you most comfortable and assert it firmly. 'I'd feel better if we split the bill, please,' 'I had a nice time, but I'd like to think about it overnight and let you know tomorrow if I want to do it again.' Notice if he can respect your boundaries.

Work out during the date if you are feeling physically attracted and interested in exploring anything physical. We all bring all sorts of variation into each and every dating encounter we have. Our experience of any one date is influenced by factors including: our relationship history, our stress / wellness levels and current emotional state, our personality, our expectations – what you think you "should" do or feel at a certain time. So, if you aren't feeling physically attracted to him at first, but you like hanging out with him ... great! That would be a good hint to keep hanging out with him, but don't be sexual yet.

How to do this practically? Be honest, uncritical, non-defensive and remember, you do not need to give excuses – as much as our brains may struggle to understand, there may be no rational reason for you to feel like this! Just keep him in touch with where you are at: '*I really love hanging out with you but I'm not feeling ready to be sexual with you right now.*'

After the date, think about whether you have any curiosity about him on any level. Would there be any positive feeling if he were to ask you out again. Make the decision as if it were a new friend who was interested in catching up with you again. It is not like you're trying to decide whether or not to marry the guy, so you don't have to agonize over it. If being asked out by him again would give you a smile, then tell him you had a nice time and you'd like to see him again. If the offer of another date would have you inwardly groaning, then either leave it, or tell him that you had a nice time, but you don't think you have enough in common. Treat him as you would like to be treated, whatever that means for you.

'I hate it when a guy sends a rejection text … I know it's probably the grown-up thing to do but it's just so awkward! And it's not as if I hadn't guessed he wasn't into it when he didn't reach out again, or he delayed his replies. I much prefer it just fading away, so that's what I do when I'm no longer into something … It feels much less stressful for me and there has only been one time when a guy didn't get the hint. I told him outright then, but I still prefer it the other way.' – Lea, 36 years old.

MANAGING AVOIDANCE

Are you the type of person who every New Year promises yourself you will begin dating only to download a dating app, freak out, and delete it? Then this plan is for you! It's based on the idea of graded exposure, a technique which has been proven to reduce anxiety and build confidence. You don't need to do all of these steps, if you feel ready to move on to the next, be my guest! However, if you go too far for yourself, and end up avoiding again, go back down to the most recent step you could do.

Step 1: Download a "least-effort" dating app like Tinder and put up one or two photos. Commit to two minutes of liking everyone in your deck every day for a week. You don't have to message them or reply to any messages you get.

Step 2: Delete the app and restart. Commit to two minutes of liking everyone in your deck *and* have a cut and paste "Hey, how has your week been?" message ready to send out to every match you get. You don't have to continue the conversations beyond this.

Step 3: Delete the app and restart. Commit to two minutes of liking everyone in your deck, start things off with your conversation starter, and agree with yourself that you will respond to any responses you get in a tit-for-tat way for a week (you can set aside a certain time each day to do this). You don't have to meet up with anyone and if anyone gets lewd, you can delete the match.

Step 4: Delete the app and restart. Commit to two minutes of liking people who meet your "fit in with friends" criteria and are within 10km from you, in your 5–10-year age bracket. If you have gotten through your two minutes and haven't liked at least 10 guys, you are being too picky – do another two minutes and be more generous.

Step 5: Continue with Step 4 every day, and add the task of starting conversations with any matches and responding to any messages. You don't have to have your phone with you 24/7, just pick a suitable time of the day (e.g. when you're on the bus home from work) and do it then.

Step 6: Once you have had a week's worth of chat, ask any matches left for a coffee! Remind yourself, this is just practice, these guys may not even be interested in meeting, and if one of them is, he'll probably be as nervous as you. Set the meeting time *soon* so you don't stew on it too much. And make it casual – an after-work drink or similar, so that you don't go to too much effort.

Step 7: Continue with the plan for as long as you need, until you lose your fear of dating. Usually once you've been on 10 dates your anxiety about the whole process is *much* less intense. You may even begin to date because you like it, and you will certainly be in a better position to actually become attracted to, and interested in a guy, rather than just sitting there wishing for the ordeal to be over with!

MANAGING ANXIETY

We all know what it's like to overthink things after a date. Did I talk too much? Did we have enough in common? Did he seem interested in me? In some ways, having some obsessive thinking after we've met someone may even be a good sign – it means our serotonin has dropped, which indicates that at least we have sufficient interest in him!

The difficulty occurs when we become overly obsessive to the point that we focus on ridding ourselves of anxiety and getting the sweet relief from him contacting us. Really, we should be enjoying the growth and connection as it naturally unfolds. In our efforts to make ourselves feel better, we are feeding our love-drug-addicted brain, and could run the risk of disrespecting our date's boundaries (expressed or not) and pushing him away.

There is no such thing as "too needy" because there is no such thing as a person without needs. My teacher, Stan Tatkin, always joked that when we get married what we should be vowing is: 'I promise to take you as my burden.'

Remember, your feelings are yours. They come from *your body*. It doesn't matter if they were provoked by the behavior of someone else, they are *your responsibility* to manage. When a single woman is called "too needy" it will usually be because: her date has very different needs in a relationship; he feels pressured to meet her needs beyond his willingness to do so; or he feels blamed when her needs aren't being met.

So, before you send that next text (or walk by his workplace again, hoping to "accidentally" run into him), read this first:

Do Contact Him If:

- The contact is motivated by feelings of excitement, curiosity, attraction, interest

- You genuinely want to hear how his day / week has been going

- You genuinely want to hear his opinion about something

- You want to share what has been going on in your world with him

- You want to invite him to something, because you are interested in seeing him again

- You want to give him some information that you think will be useful to him

- If contacting him is done with respect for what you know about him and his preferences

- If you would contact one of your closest friends in a similar way

Don't Contact Him If:

- The contact is fueled by feelings of anxiety and insecurity

- You initiate the contact to quell feelings of jealousy – wanting to know what he is doing, who he is with, etc.

- You initiate the contact purely to get him to respond so that you can put to rest thoughts about being rejected

- You catch yourself thinking up a "valid" excuse to contact him

- You have rationalized why he might not have responded to your last text / call so keep texting again, and again, and again

- What you say is angry and critical of him

- You're letting your own needs overshadow what you know about him, so you disrespect him (e.g. if you know he is busy at work during a certain time but insist on calling him during that time)

- You are ignoring his stated preferences or assertive boundaries and finding a way to do or get what you want anyway (e.g. if he tells you he needs to study and won't be able to see you one night, and you turn up at his house anyway)

'I once bought tickets to a music festival after one date with a guy who told me he was going. The festival was sold out so the tickets I bought were super expensive. I'd never been into festivals, but I wanted to look cool and I didn't want him to forget me and start hooking up with other girls while he was there! It was a disaster! The friend I took got sick on the first day, so I spent most of it trekking through the mud alone trying to look like I was having fun. I bumped into him once in the whole three days, he said he hadn't gotten my text and looked weirded out that I hadn't told him when we met up that I was going to be there too!' – Kris, 26 years old.

CHAPTER 19

DOING SINGLE WELL AFTER HEARTBREAK

No one hopes for a break-up when they begin a relationship, but with the divorce statistics so high, we can anticipate that most of us will go through a significant break-up of some kind, at some stage of our lives. Although everything you have read about Doing Single Well applies to someone recovering from a heartbreak and readjusting to single life after a long-term relationship, there are a few particular points that are worthwhile drawing out.

HEARTBREAK FEELINGS

Break-ups are experienced differently for different people, and our response to our break-up will depend on various things, including: the quality of the relationship before it ended, how well resourced we are socially, financially, and practically, our own attitude towards the break-up and what it means to us (beware of gremlins!), any pre-existing relationship trauma, and the circumstances of the break-up.

Break-up feelings are some of the most intense feelings we can feel. They can be overwhelming and disabling. We can feel a multitude of emotions which come and go randomly, such as sadness, loneliness, emptiness, anger, and despair. Most people feel they are on an "emotional rollercoaster" and will say that they can wake up feeling okay one morning only to feel awful the next.

Brain scans of heartbroken people have shown that heartbreak activates similar areas of the brain to those that get activated when we experience physical pain. We also will experience physical symptoms during heartbreak such as:

- Exhaustion, low energy, and lethargy

- Insomnia (sleeping too little) or hypersomnia (sleeping too much) and upsetting dreams

- Loss of appetite or overeating

- Muscle tightness and weakness

- Body aches and pains

- Restlessness and inability to sit still

- Nausea or a "hollow stomach"

- Indigestion and diarrhea

- Headaches

- Shortness of breath

- Palpitations / tightness in the chest

- Throat constriction

'It would have been easier if he had died! At least then I wouldn't have to live with the fact he has chosen not to be with me! I wouldn't have had to worry about bumping into him with his new girlfriend and think about her moving in to our house.' – Bec, 29 years old.

The experience of heartbreak is actually very similar to the experience of grief. We grieve the death of the relationship. Like in the Kubler Ross (1969) model of grief it can, but does not always have to, involve the following stages. These stages can occur in any order and can recur throughout the heartbreak process.

1. Denial: Not believing it is really over, thinking your ex will change his mind.

2. Anger: Lashing out at him and hating on ourselves. 'How can you do this to me?'

3. Bargaining: Feeling hopeful and trying to negotiate an alternative outcome. 'If I can just show him how fun I am, maybe he'll come back.'

4. Depression: Sadness and despair, low motivation and the desire to isolate ourselves. 'Without him I just can't be bothered.'

5. Acceptance: A feeling of calm where your emotions once again become stable. Thinking and talking about the relationship and your ex does not leave you feeling overly upset. 'It will be okay.'

Most people who are heartbroken will experience obsessive, uncontrollable thoughts about their relationship, ranging from what caused the break-up, to how they might be able to fix things. Each time a thought appears, it interrupts us, reopens our wounds, and reactivates our emotional pain. Brain studies have shown that heartbreak activates the same mechanisms in the brain that get activated when addicts are withdrawing from substances like cocaine and opioids, and the obsessiveness we first felt when we were falling in love can therefore recur at the end of the relationship.

In general, it doesn't matter how long we were in the relationship, if we had very strong feelings for our partner at some stage, we will be heartbroken by the break-up. Feelings in general are not rational, so we can experience heartbreak even if we weren't always happy in our relationship. All that is required is that our brain has experienced the love and / or attachment drugs at some stage.

Breaking up from our first love is generally thought to be the most painful heartbreak experience. But it doesn't really seem to matter how many times we've experienced heartbreak; in severe cases a broken heart can create a sustained type of stress which constitutes an emotional trauma. Risk factors for developing a trauma reaction include:

- Previous relationship trauma and insecure attachment
- Biological differences in how our brains process stress hormones
- If the break-up was a surprise or involved a betrayal
- Being left feeling peeling powerless and helpless
- Not understanding the "whys"
- Not having been able to express our point of view
- Leftover feelings of shame and self-blame

Even if we aren't heartbroken, break-ups can be difficult due to the change in our circumstances, potential change in social supports, any underlying gremlins that get activated, and any acrimony that might occur.

Because of the multiplicity of what your break-up might involve, I won't attempt to cover the issue comprehensively here. Instead I will focus on a few points that I've found have helped women adjust healthily to a break-up and come to Do Single Well. If you are really struggling with your own break-up, please do seek counseling. There are also plenty of amazing books on it. My personal favorite is *It's Called a Break-up Because It's Broken* (2009) by Greg Behrendt and Amiira Ruotola-Behrendt.

BE SELFISH

There are no prizes for being the most gracious woman to have ever gone through a break-up. No one will applaud us for giving him all our money, or all our shared friends. If we are the ones who have been rejected, our first and top priority must be giving ourselves what we need emotionally. He got to choose the timing of the break-up, and might have been thinking about it and emotionally processing it for a long time. We therefore owe it to ourselves to take our time to emotionally catch up. This means that wherever we have his cooperation, or the power to enforce it, we need to do things our own way.

For example:

- If you want to stay in your (shared) place, ask him to move out.

- If you want to get rid of his stuff ASAP, ask him to pick it up.

- If you are not ready to divide shared stuff (beyond the essentials he needs to live), tell him so, and set a date when you would be willing to revisit the issue.

- If you want to go to an event you were both invited to, or bought tickets for, and don't want him there, tell him.

- If you don't want to hear from him, tell him so.

- If you want to talk about it, try to insist on it.

- You get a say in how and when to tell the kids.

- You get a say in how and when the kids get introduced to any new partners.

In some cases, if we ask assertively (using the "I statements" we spoke about in Chapters 11 and 17) our exes will accommodate what we need. Even though they chose to break up, many people's exes will still be feeling badly for any hurt inflicted, and will have some sadness that the relationship is over. They will want to cooperate to make the process as smooth as possible. Cooperation is ideal if you can achieve it, and recovery can occur far more quickly and smoothly if you can both be fair and cooperative.

However, break-ups can bring out the worst in people. Particularly if your ex was not very good at taking responsibility, being empathic, or collaborating with you during the relationship, the chances are he might not willingly give you any power in the break-up.

When we feel disempowered and out of control of our own lives, we don't cope well. When we go through a traumatic break-up, we can feel shocked, helpless, lost, and vulnerable. An important part of any healing after trauma is reclaiming what power we do have. In a break-up this can mean anything from refusing to keep his dirty secrets, to taking him to court, if needed. With the exceptions outlined below, I encourage you to use whatever power you have to get what you need.

For example, 'I need you to pick up your things' can become 'If you don't pick up your things by Friday I will be donating them to charity' if needs be. Keep in mind that we only have power in a situation where we can implement a consequence that is meaningful to him if he fails to cooperate with what we need. 'If you insist on going to our friend's wedding despite me asking you not to, I will be telling everyone about your gambling addiction' is only powerful if he cares about whether people know about his gambling addiction.

A lot of women I speak to will sacrifice what they need in the hope of keeping their ex onside. They hope that if they are generous now, they are more likely to keep their ex amenable to them, avoid conflict, and receive more collaborative efforts later (e.g. on issues such as financial settlements and childcare). I don't recommend this. If your ex was a fair and collaborative person during the relationship, he will maintain his integrity and fairness throughout the break-up process. If your ex never demonstrated these qualities, and his decisions were more based on what he needed or his impulses in the moment, his decision making in the break-up will remain selfish and impulsive. No amount of sacrificing your needs will help this. With this type of person, we don't earn "credits" for generosity to be used at a later date, because their decisions aren't made based on reason or reciprocity.

'I went to so much effort to accommodate him when we first broke up. I gave him access to the kids whenever he wanted. Anything in the house he wanted to take with him was his. I accepted without complaint that he wouldn't pay child-support some weeks or would change his plans to pick up the children at the last minute. I had hoped that by doing this he would see how fair and reasonable I was being, and when it came to the settlement, would agree to allow me to stay in the house so the kids wouldn't have to change schools. I should have known better. He always did exactly what he wanted, and this was no exception.' – Molly, 42 years old.

When implementing consequences, we also need to do so with integrity and fairness. Keep in mind, we resort to assigning consequences for uncollaborative behavior in order to ensure that we can get what we need, rather than to punish him. We need to strike the right balance and not be a doormat, nor a bully. This means not doing anything that we can't feel proud of in the future, when all our hurt and angry feelings have resolved. Make sure any consequences you think up are logical and appropriate , e.g. 'Pick up your things by 11am today or I'll donate them' is not realistic nor fair if you haven't given him prior warning. Similarly, no matter what hurt you have sustained, being hurt is no excuse for the following:

- Abuse: Don't yell, name call, emotionally abuse him, or physically attack him.

- Defamation: No lying to others; you don't need to keep his dirty secrets, but do stick to the truth of the situation.

- Involving the kids: You can't use his access to them, or threaten their relationship with him to get what you want.

- Violating his human rights: If you can in some way prevent him from accessing money, shelter, food, employment, safety, etc. don't.

DOING SINGLE WELL: REDISCOVERING YOURSELF

Part of being in any long-term relationship means that we will have "lost" parts of ourselves due to the need to accommodate our partner's preferences. Hopefully we haven't crossed our own boundaries and the compromises we've made were made with willingness! Even so, reclaiming our own life and doing things all our own way again is an important part of rediscovering ourselves.

Try these two exercises:

1. Make a list of the things you started doing in order to accommodate your ex-partner. This can include things as small as "buying smooth peanut butter" to things as big as "buying a house in the suburbs." Make a plan of how you are going to adjust back to your own preferred way of being, then make actioning it a priority wherever possible.

2. Imagine that in six months' time you will bump into your ex in the street and have a conversation. In this imaginary world you will get to tell him how amazing and fabulous your life has become and how you have flourished since the break-up. What sorts of things do you wish you could say? Have you been traveling? Had a wardrobe revamp? Enrolled in a course? Learned the guitar? Make a list of all the things you wish you would be able to say about what you have done and then apply yourself to doing them!

HAVE YOUR SAY

Wherever possible, we need to be able to talk through and understand the break-up. Whether we agree with him or not, knowing what went wrong and how it happened according to him will help us process it and put it to rest. Similarly, sharing our perspective: how we feel, what we needed from him that he didn't give us (in the relationship or in the break-up), and also what we appreciated about the relationship is important.

Ideally your ex will be open to having these conversations with you to help you come to terms with his decision. In this case prepare yourself by:

- Writing out a list of questions: This can help if you are concerned that your emotions will overwhelm you and you won't be able to think clearly.

- Agree on specific days and times to talk about it: It is not helpful to pepper your ex with questions at all hours, he will need to be in the right headspace to manage such a difficult conversation too.

- Don't become blaming or shaming: Using one of the "Four horsemen" (Gottman, 2011) is one of the quickest ways to kill your chance at getting the information you need to get your head clear about what happened. Talking through the break-up in the presence of a counselor is a good option if you are worried about the conversation being derailed.

- Keep revisiting it: Continue to book meetings with him to talk about it until you have no questions left to answer, or until the conversation becomes circular.

- Draw a line: Once you have all the information you can get, it is then time to end the contact and take space to heal.

If your ex is not willing to talk it out with you then please do avail yourself of your friends. Yes, we will be repetitive and need to talk about it over and over. Yes, we will be emotional. But that is what friends are for! It is a sign of intimacy and trust that we feel close enough to our friends to ask them for help at such a difficult time. As a consequence, they will feel closer to us, and they'll feel more able to ask us for help through their own challenges later, if we've opened up to them.

Some friends are better than others at knowing what to do with emotional issues. We need friends who are willing to just hear us out and offer us kindness and support. We need friends who are willing to go out with us to help us forget our worries for a time. We don't need friends who are going to sympathize with our ex, gossip about us behind our back, be critical of us and how we are coping, or refuse to talk about our break-up. We need to make sure we pick the right friends.

Even when we pick the right friends, we will need to guide them as to what we need from them. Most friends will do the best that they can and offer us the support that they would want to receive if they were in our shoes. However, we are not them, and what we need will change day-by-day, so it's important to clue them in if they are off track.

In addition to telling your story to your friends it can also be helpful to: begin a journal of your thoughts, write some "unsent letters" to your ex, or talk to a counselor to help you process the break-up as quickly and kindly as you can. Remember that healing comes from expressing your truth and giving an outlet to all your emotions.

The beauty about unsent letters is that they will always stay unsent! Like in your journaling, there is no need to be balanced, to take accountability, or to be diplomatic. Journaling and unsent letters are the perfect forum for us to give ourselves permission to be as nasty and as unkind as we can manage to be! Of course, we won't always feel angry, and want to lash out, and it is perfectly okay for you to write a variety of different unsent letters or journal entries to express the multitude of your emotions. Have a look at this template of the sorts of things you may want to address in your writing:

DOING SINGLE WELL: UNSENT LETTER

Hi (Insert ex's name),

When you told me you wanted to end our relationship I felt ...

My dreams for us had always been ...

That you no longer shared those dreams or wanted to participate in our relationship meant to me ...

What I needed from you that I never received in the relationship was ...

What I needed from you that I never received in the break-up was ...

Although we had many good times including ....

We also had many bad times including ...

Although I fell in love with these qualities of yours ...

It is for the best that our relationship has ended because you have shown me that you also have these qualities ...

I acknowledge that I could have done these things better ...

However, in the end, our relationship has ended because you were unwilling or unable to work through things with me and put in the time and effort needed to get us back on track. This shows me that either we are too different to make a relationship work, or that you (or "we" if you feel you share some of the blame) don't have the relationship skills needed to make a relationship work.

Because I could never count on you to give me / provide for my (unmet needs ...) I'm now going to do this (insert how you are going to meet your own needs from now on).

Your ex

(Sign your name)

To contact or not to contact?

Although our goal is to eventually lead separate and independent lives, I don't think the issue of cutting contact is as black and white as you might read elsewhere.

I don't think we should cut contact out of pride, to cover up our vulnerability and hurt, or because we are embarrassed that we still feel love for him. Yes, our ex has said he doesn't want to be with us anymore, but that doesn't mean he will be unsympathetic or critical of the pain we feel as a consequence of that. Nor should we be unsympathetic or critical of ourselves! Of course we will feel intense pain after a break-up, and have the impulse to reach out to him. This is a normal part of having been attached to him. We should be proud of our capacity to feel the pain we are in because it speaks of our capacity to love.

We need to try to accept and allow space to experience all our feelings, including our hopefulness, hurt, anger, and sadness.

We need to try to meet our own needs and care for ourselves through those feelings just as we would with any feelings we have (see Chapter 8).

In addition to meeting our own needs, break-ups are perfect times to enlist the support of friends. Because we will feel abandoned and alone as a result of the rejection, having the support of friends will remind you that there are people that care, and are always there for you. Enlisting a "break-up buddy" to contact instead of contacting him when we feel that impulse can be helpful. If he broke up the relationship, he is essentially saying he no longer wants to be the one we turn towards to get our emotional needs met, and it is important that once we have a handle on the break-up, we try to respect that.

However, it is overly mean and unhelpful to beat ourselves up if we slip up and contact him. Be it a drunk-dial or an impulsive "missing you" text, these things will no doubt happen, and don't have to mean you are a loser or a lost-cause. My years treating clients in therapy have shown me that our emotional brains can be much more powerful than our rational brains – that's why I have a job! So, if your emotional brain overpowers your rational brain during a break-up, it is not a character flaw, just part of being in a human body.

You can even have compassion for your angry feelings; they too are very normal. However, being angry does not make it okay to behave aggressively or abusively. If you find yourself overly impulsive and prone to hostile texts or calls, the compassionate thing to do, both for yourself and your ex, is to block his number or email, or give your phone to friends when going out so that you can't be tempted to act out abusively. Try instead to use an unsent letter to help you express and process your anger.

There are times I will actively encourage or support clients in re-contacting their exes. You've already read how I support having as many conversations as we need in order to understand and process the break-up. Even if this is not possible there is still an argument for exposing ourselves to contact with our ex in order to heal any unresolved trauma.

When we experience a traumatic break-up we develop a host of strong feelings in response to thoughts, memories, and the triggers that remind us of the relationship and our exes. Some people respond to this by trying to shut down their feelings, not talk about or think about the break-up, and shut their ex out of their life in order to avoid the pain. However, as with anything we avoid, this can stop us getting further information to change any faulty beliefs.

An arachnophobe (someone who is afraid of spiders) will need to play with real spiders to change their belief that spiders will attack them. No amount of intellectual "knowing" that they are being silly will change the fear in the way that experience does. Similarly, we need to activate the break-up emotions and bring up our faulty beliefs in a real-life, experiential way to have the right conditions to re-process and re-understand our traumatic break-up experience.

By far the most common trauma in break-ups is the basic trauma of being rejected. Most people who can't move on from a break-up will focus on that rejection and how they were "not good enough" (thank you, gremlin!) to keep their partner's love. Yet, we all know no one is perfect (which means your ex had flaws too) and that it takes two people to make a relationship work.

Further contact with your ex, with the mindset of trying to see his flaws and the reasons why he wasn't good enough (either as a person for you, or in terms of his relationship skills) can help re-empower you. Just as with being rejected early on in dating, we need to remember that break-ups are just someone realizing an incompatibility before you did, or someone demonstrating their lack of relationship skills.

If contacting your ex sounds horrible to you, or is impossible, there are certainly other ways to activate your break-up feelings and beliefs. Unsent letters might do this. Emotional conversations with wise friends or seeing a skillful counselor might do this. Getting into a new relationship might do this. However, if it is possible, contacting your ex is not such a bad idea, so long as you have the right mindset.

If you don't understand the break-up, or have developed faulty beliefs from the break-up (thank you, gremlins and man myths!) further contact with your ex could be a fast way of giving you the new information you need to change your unhelpful thinking. If the relationship has been over for a while and you've found yourself yearning for the past relationship, forgetting the things that broke you up, that might also be a good time to get in touch with him. Hopefully seeing him will remind you.

There are three key questions to help you make your decision about whether further contact with your ex will be useful to you:

1. What is the likelihood I will learn anything new, or be reminded of what went wrong, by contacting him?

2. Will I be able to keep a critical mind and go searching for information to challenge my unhelpful thinking if I get in touch?

3. When I've contacted him in the past, did it help me see things more clearly and help me emotionally to move on from the relationship?

'I'd held a candle for my ex for years after the break-up. We had had a five-year-long relationship and I still didn't understand why he chose to end it. I'd thought that I wasn't good enough as a partner. When we caught up for coffee a year ago it was the best thing I could have done. All he spoke about was his work and his career goals, how exhausted he was, and how under-appreciated he felt by his boss ... it was so familiar! He barely mentioned his current partner, except to call her "needy" and I ended up feeling sorry for her. It couldn't have been more clear: with his entire focus on his work, no relationship would ever be the priority .' – Anne, 32 years old.

OUTSOURCE IMPORTANT DECISION MAKING

Because we are under stress and experiencing heightened emotionality as a result of a heartbreak, we are not in the best place to be making decisions. Important decisions, from drastic hairstyle changes to agreeing on a financial settlement need to at least be run by close, honest friends and family members, if not run by experienced professionals. Most women will try to avoid legal battles with their ex if they can as it can be costly and time consuming.

However, a good family lawyer has the experience you don't have in break-ups and will be able to tell you what is reasonable to agree to, and what isn't. Remember, just as consulting a medical specialist doesn't necessarily mean you'll end up in hospital, getting legal advice does not necessarily mean you'll end up in the court room. Therefore, if there is any doubt that you are acting with your own best interests in mind, please do seek legal advice. This could occur in situations such as:

- If you have a history of self-sacrifice, being conflict avoidant, and trying to please your partner

- If you've been blind-sided by the break-up

- If you feel pressured by your ex to make fast decisions

- If your ex has a history of being controlling and wanting things all his way

DON'T INVOLVE THE KIDS

Lots of women stay in bad relationships too long in order to protect their children. However, it is far better for children *if* their parents separate, rather than living in a conflict-ridden house if that means they aren't exposed to further conflict. As such, even if your ex-partner does not play by these rules, try to abide by the following:

- Tell your kids that you still love them, and that the break-up has nothing to do with them. You will be there for them no matter what.

- Don't criticize their father to them or in their earshot. If he behaves badly then speak of the behavior *not* the person, 'I'm not happy that Daddy didn't call you when he said he would.' *Not* 'Your Daddy is a self-absorbed loser!'

- Don't hide your distress, normalize it, 'Mummy is feeling sad because of all the changes but I'll be okay.'

- Don't emotionally lean on your children – show them you can care for your own feelings. So don't ask them for hugs when you feel upset, don't ask them to stay home to keep you company, etc.

- Don't ask them to choose who they want to see and when; tell them what is going to happen based on the agreements you have made with your ex.

- Be available to listen to their feelings and thoughts, have a regular "chat time" (e.g. bedtime) to encourage them to express what is coming up for them.

- Don't ask your children to keep secrets from your ex (unless it would be dangerous not to).

- Don't ask your children for information about your ex, and if they tell you things that you didn't know, don't make a big deal of it in front of them.

- Seek counseling for your children if their mood of behavior changes in a significant way.

WHEN TO BEGIN DATING

There are no rules about when is a good time to begin dating, so don't listen to anyone else's views over listening to your own needs and feelings. Of course, break-ups can be busy times and many women need to focus on the practical business of breaking up (moving house, settling finances, custody arrangements, etc.) before they can think about meeting someone new. However, prioritizing self-care is important throughout the break-up process, particularly if it looks as if it is going to be a long, drawn-out one, and dating can certainly be part of this self-care.

Some women find it useful to date almost immediately after a break-up to beat the "not good enough" gremlins or challenge the "there's no one like him" man myths. This is great, there is no better way to remind yourself that you are still attractive and desirable than having other people attracted to you! There is no better way to see that your ex may not be as good as you have made him out to be, than being treated beautifully by someone else!

A lot of women find that even though they might meet some lovely guys, they just don't seem to be able to fall in love with them while they are grieving their past relationship. This is perfectly normal and what is behind the "rebound" relationship concept. Because of the way our nervous system and neurochemicals work (see Chapters 13 and 14) we can't often fall in love with someone new if grieving the old relationship is depleting our stores of the neurotransmitters needed to fall in love. This is not a reason to stop dating necessarily, we just need to have reasonable expectations of what we might feel, and not let our lack of feelings trick us into believing the "no one like him" man myth!

Some women find that dating straightaway makes them more depressed and miserable because they are in a headspace of "selective negative thinking" (Chapter 4) and therefore can't find fun and enjoy their dates. In this case, it is wise to take a break from dating and put more work into healthily processing the break-up. However, if you haven't tried dating, don't assume this is how you'll feel. It is actually far more common that women avoid dating for the wrong reasons (see Chapter 9) than put off dating for the right ones.

Don't Date:

- To make him jealous

- For fear of "being left on the shelf"

- To avoid negative feelings e.g. loneliness

- Because others have told you that you should (if you are actually happy being single)

Do Date:

- If you are curious

- If you have some gremlins or man myths you need to overcome

- If you have always dreamed of being in a partnership

- If the only reason you aren't is one of the reasons we covered in Chapter 9

MANAGING HOSTILITY

Although we would all like to feel we can get through break-ups as the grown-ups we are, the flood of horrible feelings on top of the communication and relationship issues that may have caused the break-up in the first place will generally mean that some hostility is inevitable.

We need to do what we can to manage our anger and resentment without acting out in a hostile way towards our partner. Even though he hurt us, we should not use him as an emotional punching bag. To help with this, try: journaling, writing unsent letters, establishing healthy boundaries, giving yourself what you need as a priority, and talking it out with friends or a counselor.

However, the important thing to realize about anger is that it can be an automatic response from our nervous system if we feel attacked. This means that no matter how well we process the break-up and gain clarity and acceptance of what went wrong, if we keep feeling attacked, and criticized, or our boundaries keep being violated, we will likely experience anger and resentment. We will also be more likely to respond with hostility as the situation escalates.

As such, it is important that we don't let ourselves be bullied by an ex-partner. If you continue to receive nasty texts, phone calls, or emails, set a clear boundary and escalate the consequences if he does not respect it.

'I will not be responding to any more communications that contain hostility.'

Can lead to:

'Because you continue to send me hostile emails / texts I will be blocking your address / number.'

Blocking contact with someone who will not respect our boundaries needs to be done as quickly as possible to begin our moving on from the relationship. Keep in mind that if he is behaving in this way after we have given him fair warning, he is acting from impulse and emotion, and is not being reasonable or rational. Even if he apologizes when he calms down, we can't rely on any promises he makes to change his behavior, until his emotional control changes. This may happen in time, but if he was always impulsive and quick to anger and blame, then don't rely on it. Protect yourself and him by blocking him.

If you can't completely cut him out of your life due to children, make sure you arrange any contact to occur where you can feel the abuse will be minimized. Telling him that you are blocking him and instructing him to direct any communication he needs to make about the arrangements with the children to a relative or friend can be a good option. Arranging the exchange of children in a public space (e.g. at the preschool grounds or on the street in the presence of others) can also help.

The less chance he gets to vent on you the more likely he will move on. However, you do need to be consistent. Don't give in and let him vent to you. Don't respond to nasty emails / texts out of pity, guilt, or exhaustion. Like the slot machine we spoke about in Chapter 15, this "intermittent reinforcement" will actually just ensure that his bad behavior continues for longer.

Please also keep in mind that if you feel intimidated or unsafe, even if he has never threatened you physically, you may have a case to go to the police and seek official intervention. Emotional abuse is just as damaging as physical abuse and needs to be taken just as seriously.

DEALING WITH THE "OTHER WOMAN"

Few people leave a long-term relationship without at least an idea of someone else in mind. As such, sooner or later we will have to cope with another woman in our ex's (and our kids') lives. If he left for someone else, it can be so tempting to direct all our anger onto the "other woman" and make her out to be the villain. However, your ex was the one who broke his commitment to you, and therefore the responsibility for your broken heart lies with him.

Many affairs are "innocently done" in that most people who cheat on their partners don't set out to cheat. I generally find an affair occurs due to the combination of ignorance, liking, attraction, and proximity. Your ex was likely to have liked this woman, been attracted to her, had the opportunity to see her regularly, and been ignorant that this repeated contact with deepening intimacy would cause him to fall in love. Once this process begins it would have become easy for him to open intimacy "windows" for her while erecting intimacy "walls" with you (NOT "Just Friends": Rebuilding Trust and Recovering Your Sanity After Infidelity by Glass and Staheli, 2007 is a great book if you need more on the subject). Add a drop of alcohol and then sexual contact is inevitable.

This is not to excuse your ex's behavior – he should have come to you to talk through what was happening. You could have made a plan together for him to set some boundaries with this other woman, and emotionally reconnect with you. However, if you are thinking that there was something wrong with you, or big problems in your relationship that caused the affair, don't. Although sometimes there are unaddressed issues in a relationship that precede an affair, this is not necessarily the case.

Although you may feel like the "loser" of this situation, you are just as worthy as this other woman. He may be in love with her, and he may have chosen to be with her, but that does not mean she is objectively more attractive, more intelligent, more funny, more caring, more anything than you. Unfortunately, his brain is on drugs. Unfortunately, he is thinking that his chances of happiness are better with her. I'm not saying this is never the truth of the matter. However, in the haze of new love we don't often see clearly, and her flaws (which she will most certainly have) may not be as evident to him as yours are, given the many years you may have been together.

And that's okay. That's his problem to deal with in the months and years to come. You won't be giving in to "not good enough" gremlins or "no one like him" man myths. You won't be waiting for him to come to his senses. You will be Doing Single Well!

So, try not to make the "other woman" out to be something special, it gives her power in your mind that she doesn't deserve. Odds are she is an ordinary lady just like you. If she is here to stay and you are going to see her because of your children or shared friends, make sure you don't avoid her. Take control and meet with her as soon as you can. Approach her at that party and introduce yourself. It will be awkward for you both, but it will get easier with repetition, and it is far better than you giving up parts of your life and all of your power to avoid her.

SHARING FRIENDS

Some of the heartbreak of breaking up can actually be the losses beyond the relationship. Feeling like you have to lose his family or shared friends from your life can compound the feeling of desolation. Once again, I encourage you to seek to have it your way. Reach out to the people in your life and ask for what you would like. There are no prizes for bowing out graciously and these people may not know you care about maintaining your relationship with them unless you tell them. Not everyone will be able to meet your needs, but it can't hurt to ask.

If you care about continued contact with friends that are more "his" tell them that. Tell them how appreciative of their friendship you have been during the relationship and express your hopes that even though your relationship is over, you can still stay in touch. Better still, initiate social occasions with them!

If you don't feel comfortable with your friends having contact with your ex, then tell them that. Explain how you are feeling and how important it is for you that they have your back at this time. If they don't feel that they can cut him from their lives, then seek to understand why, and set some boundaries about how you would like them to manage situations like invitations to events and information about your ex.

It is a common experience for people that are newly single to feel abandoned by their "couple" friends. Rather than invite one or the other of a broken-up pair, the couples invite neither. If this is your experience, address it directly with the couples involved. Express what you need from them, and talk about the situations you used to enjoy that you would like to continue to be a part of. Model for them how you want your experiences with them to continue by organizing some yourself.

Remember that your ex is responsible for his own social circumstances; there is no need for you to think of his needs. It could well be that he doesn't care about contact with the people, or being invited to the occasions that you dearly miss. If he does, then it is up to your friends how they choose to manage any competing interests, and you can only respond to the decisions that they make. Ask for what you'd like. Wait for their decision. Work out if what they have chosen is still something you want to be a part of. Like any boundary issue (remember the Boundary Bagel exercise in Chapter 5?) there will be areas where you can willingly compromise and areas where you can't.

NOSTALGIA

Just because you have good memories of your ex or your time together, it doesn't mean that you aren't over the relationship. In fact, it can be a sign of good healing that you can objectively see the strengths of the relationship while not minimizing the difficulties.

Nostalgia is a sentimentality for the past, usually associated with yearning. Historian Svetlana Boym (2016) identified two types of nostalgia: "restorative" and "reflective" nostalgia. With restorative nostalgia we attempt to re-live the past in the present. When we hear "our song" on the radio we call our ex and attempt to re-live the feelings we had at that time. This can lead to feelings of pain and unfulfilled longing.

With reflective nostalgia, we accept the fact that the past is the past and we can appreciate the memories for what they are and experience the pleasure they lend to this moment without fretting over the fact that we can never actually re-live it. We can listen to "our song" and feel some pleasure from it without having to reach out to our ex.

Nostalgia will often come up at times of transition, change, and uncertainty. During periods of instability, nostalgic reminiscence can be a stabilizing force that strengthens and reassures us. It can also positively motivate us to confront our fears, take reasonable risks and tackle challenges, in the same way that feelings of anticipation can.

The only caution we need to be mindful of is that our brain is wired to remember "peak" experiences more than the mundane ones and so we can have an overly rose-tinted view of the past when looking through the lens of nostalgia. However, so long as we don't romanticize our past relationships, and keep a realistic perspective on both the good and bad, nostalgia can help us integrate our past-relationship experiences into the story of our lives ensuring that no time spent in any relationship is a waste of our time.

CHAPTER 20

'I DO'

It's afternoon, on an unusually rainy February Sunday, in Sydney. I'm sitting here on my couch, my feet in my favorite cashmere bed socks with my giant cat Mr Max purring away next to me. I realize I haven't spoken a word all day and I haven't missed it at all.

Yesterday at a lunch that turned into dinner, over many bottles of wine, I was telling my gay buddies about how I was finding it difficult to end this book. The cliché ending of the single woman finding love, donning white tulle, and ecstatically reciting her wedding vows is such a dominant narrative that I've been at a loss as to how I could provide a powerful alternative.

I got my light bulb moment later that night after receiving a touching text from one of those same friends: 'Gem, we had such a great time today, it was so good seeing you. You are a deeply interesting, amazing, and inspiring woman.'

If that wasn't a declaration of love, I don't know what is!

If you are to take just one thing away about Doing Single Well, I want it to be this: You don't need a partner to have love in your life. And when your life is filled with love, you forget that you are "single." You are just you, living your awesome life.

If I am anything, I am an advocate of love. I am not against marriage or coupling. I believe in gay marriage – for those that want it – because I believe that it speaks to a society of people who are trying to love and respect all their citizens equally. It is this same love and respect that I hope single women will begin to enjoy on a cultural level.

As we discussed, love is not a fleeting feeling, but the product of many consistent actions. On a society level, these actions must be in service of reducing the singlism that is built into the very fabric of day-to-day life. While I'm relieved to see the rise of communal dining tables in restaurants, and the increased number of single-serve meal options in the supermarkets, we have a long way to go.

On a personal level, we must learn to turn the female cultural prescription of "caregiver" towards ourselves – to invest in acts of love towards ourselves as a priority. Love can come from connection with your tribe. Love can come in the form of finding purpose and meaning – loving what you do. Love can be in the creating of a home, and the daily acts of how you care for yourself. Love can come in setting boundaries, so you are not hurt by comments from the well-meaning. Love can come in cleaning up your dating, and not allowing yourself to avoid, step over your own boundaries, or settle for unavailable men. But the best kind of love, the kind that can never be lost or taken from you, is ...

the love you show yourself when you know and own your stuff, when you accept yourself completely, and live (and date, if you desire it) with authenticity.

It is this self-love and my commitment to continually getting to know and act with love towards myself that I believe makes me the satisfied single woman I am. In Gottman's 'Sound relationship house' terms: I take time to know my inner world, I have fondness and admiration for myself in all my beautiful imperfection, I turn towards my emotions and try to have my own back by prioritizing meeting my emotional needs. I take the positive perspective with myself, and work hard not to let any "not good enough" gremlins create internal conflict, and I'm committed to making my life meaningful, and fulfilling my dreams.

SINGLE WOMEN VERSION:

Create a meaningful life: Stay in touch with your values and create purpose.

Make life dreams come true: Don't put anything on hold. Make your dreams a priority now.

Create a meaningful life – Stay in touch with your values and create purpose.

Make your life dreams come true – Don't put anything on hold. Make pursuing your dreams a priority now.

Interpersonal skills – Set healthy boundaries with the well meaning, and on dates. Know who you are and give yourself permission to speak your truth, don't compromise your truth for the sake of pleasing others.

The positive perspective – Take an attitude of gratitude towards yourself and your life. Focus on the things you can enjoy. Stay active and curious when dating and in in life generally.

Turning towards yourself – Meet your own needs as you are your first priority. Take time to pay attention to your feelings and care for yourself through any negative emotions.

Fondness and admiration – Act with compassion and kindness towards yourself. Embrace your imperfections. Act like your own "best friend."

Love maps – Know yourself and your stuff, be aware of self-criticism (gremlins), man myths and unhelpful thinking and dating patterns.

Set boundaries and manage conflict: Set healthy boundaries with the well-meaning and on dates. Be assertive.

By paralleling the ingredients of satisfied single life to those that make a happy couple, I hope that the truth that has been implicit in this whole book becomes obvious: there is very little difference between the journey to having a healthy relationship with a man and the journey to Doing Single Well. Happiness has nothing to do with being part of a couple, or being single, and much more to do with investing effort into being self-aware, self-fulfilled, accepting of yourself, and acting with love and kindness in all things.

It occurs to me that staying true to yourself in this way, whether you enter into a relationship or remain single, is just as great an achievement as fulfilling any marital vows. It is a competitive, superficial, and perfectionistic world we live in. It's so easy to get sucked into having an affair with self-criticism, worry about the future, or ruminate on what we "should" have been, done or achieved. There will always be someone prettier. There will always be someone younger. There will always be someone smarter. There will always be someone more successful. But there will never be someone just like you.

Saying 'I do' to loving yourself, and staying committed to the unique and beautiful individual you are, is one of the worthiest goals I can imagine. Such a promise is deserving of all the fluff and fanfare, confetti and commotion, of the most sensational of weddings. So, why not throw an amazing party to celebrate yourself if that appeals? There is no reason at all why you should wait to find "the one"... you've always been her anyway!

Also take the time to write your personal vows to yourself describing the kind of life partner that you are committed to being. Write them up beautifully and put them on the bathroom mirror, or frame them on the wall, as a daily reminder of your promise to yourself, and please do share them with us @doingsinglewell

Enjoy yourself!

Gemma

GEMMA'S VOWS TO HERSELF

I promise to love myself, to laugh at my mistakes, smile fondly at my imperfections, and celebrate the parts of my life that I haven't yet mastered.

I promise to care for myself, to never let myself feel deprived because I haven't been thoughtful enough to buy myself groceries. To never let myself feel exhausted because I haven't listened to my energy levels and stayed too late at work.

I promise to protect myself from the toxic people in my life. To set boundaries and spend my time with the people, and doing the activities, that fill me with joy.

I promise to be bold and express myself exuberantly, uncaring of the approval of others. To follow my whims without worry and dare to dream big.

I promise to be generous. To treat myself like a princess and not skimp on anything "because it's just me."

I promise to be open and curious. To remain conscious of myself, my changing feelings and needs, and continue to deepen my knowledge of myself and my stuff at every opportunity.

I promise to have a passionate marriage to myself, to be my own soulmate and live life in vibrant color, full of wonder, love, and laughter.

ACKNOWLEDGMENTS

To all the women who have shared their stories with me so generously (and without any fear of vulnerability). This book is for you.

To the magnificent female mentors I've had in my own life – women who continue to encourage and inspire me: Fiona Ann Papps, Larraine Hall, and Marie-Pierre Cleret.

To the best man and teacher I know, Michael Yapko. A truly remarkable human in what seems to be a truly remarkable partnership with his wife Diane – If I manage to create a relationship like that, there may just be a *Doing Relationships Well* sequel!

To my mum and dad who gave me my "stuff" both helpful and questionably helpful, but without which I wouldn't be on the journey I am today – love you. Also to my Uncle John and Aunty Helen who helped me with the family history.

To my friends who have read drafts and listened to my soap-boxing. Particularly Amy, Katey, Lizzy, Liv, Emma, Phil, Ross, David, Josh, and Adam (well, having a lot of friends is important to Doing Single Well!), to Danny – who is always there for me, and Shane who gave me the inspiration I needed to write the last chapter.

To Chris and the Trigger crew for their enthusiasm, support, and the important work that they do, giving a voice to mental health issues.

(To my cat Mr Max a gentle giant of a rescue cat and my faithful writing buddy – adopt don't shop!)

Finally, to you, the reader. May you get what you need to "Do Single Well" and know that your purchase helps others get what they need, as contributing proceeds support the global mental health charity, The Shaw Mind Foundation.

If you found this book interesting ...
why not read this next?

Body Image Problems
& Body Dysmorphic Disorder

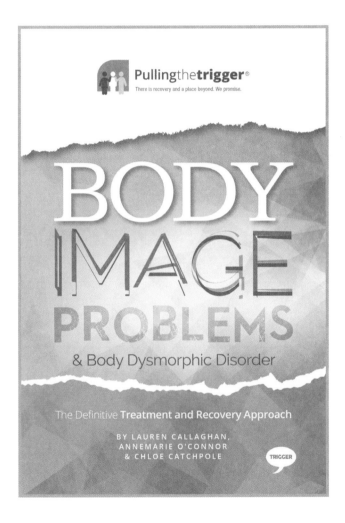

This unique and inspiring book provides simple yet highly effective self-help methods to help you overcome your body image concerns and Body Dysmorphic Disorder (BDD).

REFERENCES

AUSTEN, J. (2009). *Pride and Prejudice*. New York, Middleton Classics Publishing.

BEHRENDT, G., & RUOTOLA-BEHRENDT, A. (2006). *It's Called a Breakup Because It's Broken: The Smart Girl's Breakup Buddy*. London, HarperElement.

BROWN, B. (2010). *The Gifts of Imperfection: Let Go of Who You Think You're Supposed to Be and Embrace Who You Are*. Center City, MN Hazelden.

BUSS, D. M. (1989). Sex differences in human mate preferences: Evolutionary hypotheses tested in 37 cultures. *Behavioral and Brain Sciences*. 12(1), 1 -14.

BUSS, D. M. et al. (1990). International preferences in selecting mates: a study in 37 cultures. *Journal of Cross-Cultural Psychology*, 21(1), 5–47. Universität Bielefeld. http://repositories.ub.uni-bielefeld.de/biprints/volltexte/2009/2337/.

CHAPMAN, G. (1995). *The Five Love Languages*. Chicago, IL, Northfield Publishing.

CLINE, S. (1994). *Women, Celibacy and Passion*. London, Optima.

COHEN, A. S., KALMAN, M., & VON TEESE, D. (2012). *Advanced Style*. Brooklyn, NY PowerHouse Books.

DE ANGELIS, B. (2013). *Are You the One for Me?: How to Have the Relationship You've Always Wanted*. London, Harper Element.

DEPAULO, B. M. (2007). *Singled Out: How Singles Are Stereotyped, Stigmatized, and Ignored, and Still Live Happily Ever After*. New York, St Martin's Griffin.

DEPAULO, B. M. (2015). *Marriage vs. Single Life: How Science and the Media Got it So Wrong*. CreateSpace Independent Publishing

DEPAULO, B., & MORRIS, W. (2005). TARGET ARTICLE: Singles in society and in science. *Psychological Inquiry*. 16, 57–83.

DOHERTY, W. J. (1997). *The Intentional Family: How to Build Family Ties in Our Modern World.* Reading, MA, Addison-Wesley Publishing.

DOWRICK, S. (2014). *Intimacy and Solitude.* Crows Nest, NSW, Allen & Unwin.

DUTTON, D. G, & ARON A. P. (1974). Some evidence for heightened sexual attraction under conditions of high anxiety. *Journal of Personality and Social Psychology.* 30, 510–17.

FISHER, H. E. (2010). *Why Him? Why Her?* New York, Henry Holt & Co.

FREUD, Sigmund (1912). Über die allgemeinste Erniedrigung des Liebeslebens [The most prevalent form of degradation in erotic life]. *Jahrbuch für psychoanalytische und psychopathologische Forschungen.* 4, 40–50.

GLASS, S with STAHELI, J. C. (2007). *NOT "Just Friends": Rebuilding Trust and Recovering Your Sanity After Infidelity.* New York, Simon and Schuster.

GOTTMAN, J. M., & SILVER, N. (1999). *The Seven Principles for Making Marriage Work: A Practical Guide from the Country's Foremost Relationship Expert.* Old Saybrook, Ct, Tantor Media, Inc.

GREENWOOD, J., SESHADRI, A., & YORUKOGLU, M. (2005). Engines of liberation. *Review of Economic Studies.* 72, 109–33.

HARRIS, R. (2009). *ACT with Love: Stop Struggling, Reconcile Differences, and Strengthen your Relationship with Acceptance and Commitment Therapy.* Oakland, CA, New Harbinger Publications.

HOMER. (1962). *Illiad.* Chicago, Great Books Foundation.

KING, R. (1998). *Good Loving, Great Sex: Finding Balance when your Sex Drives Differ.* Milsons Point, NSW, Arrow.

KNIGHT, S. (2016). *The Life-Changing Magic of Not Giving a F**k: How To Stop Spending Time You Don't Have Doing Things You Don't Want To Do With People You Don't Like.* London, Quercus Publishing.

LEJEUNE, C. (2007). *The Worry Trap: How to Free Yourself from Worry & Anxiety Using Acceptance and Commitment Therapy.* Oakland, CA, New Harbinger Publications.

MCGRAW, P. C. (2007). *Love Smart: Find the One You want, Fix the One You Got.* New York, Free Press.

REIS, H. T., CLARK, M. S., & HOLMES, J. G. (2004). Perceived partner responsiveness as an organizing construct in the study of intimacy and closeness. In D. J. Mashek & A. P. Aron (Eds.), *Handbook of Closeness and Intimacy* (pp. 201–25). Mahwah, NJ, Lawrence Erlbaum Associates.

SHAKESPEARE, W. (1597). *Romeo and Juliet.*

SWAMI, V. et al. (2010). The attractive female body weight and female body dissatisfaction in 26 countries across 10 world regions: Results of the International Body Project I. *Personality and Social Psychology Bulletin.* 36, 309–25.

TATKIN, S. (2012). *Wired for Love.* Oakland, New Harbinger.

TATKIN, S. (2016). *Wired for Dating: How Understanding Neurobiology and Attachment Style Can Help You Find Your Ideal Mate.* Oakland, CA, New Harbinger Publications, Inc.

TRAISTER, R. (2016). *All the Single Ladies: Unmarried Women and the Rise of an Independent Nation.* New York, Simon & Schuster.

TRIMBERGER, E. K. (2005). *The New Single Woman.* Boston, MA Beacon Press.

YAPKO, M. (2010). *Depression Is Contagious: How the Most Common Mood Disorder is Spreading Around the World and How to Stop It.* Free Pr.

WARNER, M. (1991). Introduction: Fear of a Queer Planet. Social Text; 9(4), 3–17.

WOLF, N. (1997). *Promiscuities: The Secret Struggle for Womanhood.* New York, Fawcett Columbine.

ZHANG, Y., KONG, F., ZHONG, Y., & KOU, H. (2014). *Personality manipulations: Do they modulate facial attractiveness ratings? Personality and Individual Differences.* 70, 80.

INDEX

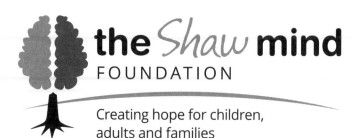

the *Shaw* mind
FOUNDATION

Creating hope for children,
adults and families

Sign up to our charity, The Shaw Mind Foundation

www.shawmindfoundation.org

and keep in touch with us; we would love to hear from you.

*Our goal is to make help and support available for every
single person in society, from all walks of life.
We will never stop offering hope. These are our promises.*

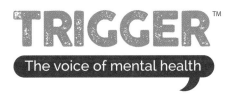

www.triggerpublishing.com

Trigger is a publishing house devoted to opening conversations about mental health. We tell the stories of people who have suffered from mental illnesses and recovered, so that others may learn from them.

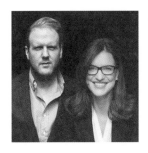

Adam Shaw is a worldwide mental health advocate and philanthropist. Now in recovery from mental health issues, he is committed to helping others suffering from debilitating mental health issues through the global charity he co-founded, The Shaw Mind Foundation. www.shawmindfoundation.org

Lauren Callaghan (CPsychol, PGDipClinPsych, PgCert, MA (hons), LLB (hons), BA), born and educated in New Zealand, is an innovative industry-leading psychologist based in London, United Kingdom. Lauren has worked with children and young people, and their families, in a number of clinical settings providing evidence based treatments for a range of illnesses, including anxiety and obsessional problems. She was a psychologist at the specialist national treatment centres for severe obsessional problems in the UK and is renowned as an expert in the field of mental health, recognised for diagnosing and successfully treating OCD and anxiety related illnesses in particular. In addition to appearing as a treating clinician in the critically acclaimed and BAFTA award-winning documentary *Bedlam*, Lauren is a frequent guest speaker on mental health conditions in the media and at academic conferences. Lauren also acts as a guest lecturer and honorary researcher at the Institute of Psychiatry Kings College, UCL.

Please visit the link below:

www.triggerpublishing.com

Join us and follow us...

@triggerpub

@Shaw_Mind

Search for us on Facebook